Enabling Rapid and Sustainable Public Health Research During Disasters

Summary of a Joint Workshop by the Institute of Medicine and the U.S. Department of Health and Human Services

Forum on Medical and Public Health Preparedness for Catastrophic Events

Board on Health Sciences Policy

Megan Reeve, Theresa Wizemann, and Bruce Altevogt,
Rapporteurs

INSTITUTE OF MEDICINE
OF THE NATIONAL ACADEMIES

THE NATIONAL ACADEMIES PRESS
Washington, D.C.
www.nap.edu

THE NATIONAL ACADEMIES PRESS • 500 Fifth Street, NW • Washington, DC 20001

NOTICE: The workshop that is the subject of this workshop summary was approved by the Governing Board of the National Research Council, whose members are drawn from the councils of the National Academy of Sciences, the National Academy of Engineering, and the Institute of Medicine.

This activity was supported by contracts between the National Academy of Sciences and the American College of Emergency Physicians; American Hospital Association; Association of State and Territorial Health Officials; Centers for Disease Control and Prevention (Contract No. 200-2011-38807, TO #30); Department of Defense (Contract No. HT0011-11-P-0186); Department of Defense, Uniformed Services University of the Health Sciences (Contract No. HT9404-12-1-0022); Department of Health and Human Services' Administration for Children and Families (Contract No. HHSP233201400153 3P); Department of Health and Human Services' National Institutes of Health: National Institute of Allergy and Infectious Diseases, National Institute of Environmental Sciences, National Library of Medicine (Contract No. HHSN26300007 [Under Base 1 #HHSN2 63201200074I]); Department of Health and Human Services' Office of the Assistant Secretary for Preparedness and Response (Contract No. HHSO100201000021P); Department of Homeland Security's Federal Emergency Management Agency (Contract No. HSFE20-13-P-0212); Department of Homeland Security, Office of Health Affairs (Contract No. HSHQDC-13-J-00384 [Under Base 1 #HSHQDC-11-D-00009]); Department of Transportation's National Highway Traffic Safety Administration (Contract No. DTNH22-10-H-00287); Department of Veterans Affairs (Contract No. 101-G09041); Emergency Nurses Association; Food and Drug Administration (Contract No. HHSF22301027T [Under Base Contract DHHS-8598]); Infectious Diseases Society of America; Martin, Blanck & Associates; Mayo Clinic; Merck Research Laboratories (Contract No. APA-2014-1666); National Association of Chain Drug Stores; National Association of County and City Health Officials; National Association of Emergency Medical Technicians; Pharmaceutical Research and Manufacturers of America; Robert Wood Johnson Foundation; Society for Disaster Medicine and Public Health; Target Corporation; Trauma Center Association of America; and United Health Foundation. The views presented in this publication do not necessarily reflect the views of the organizations or agencies that provided support for the activity.

International Standard Book Number-13: 978-0-309-31330-8
International Standard Book Number-10: 0-309-31330-9

Additional copies of this workshop summary are available for sale from the National Academies Press, 500 Fifth Street, NW, Keck 360, Washington, DC 20001; (800) 624-6242 or (202) 334-3313; http://www.nap.edu.

For more information about the Institute of Medicine, visit the IOM home page at: **www.iom.edu.**

Printed in the United States of America

The serpent has been a symbol of long life, healing, and knowledge among almost all cultures and religions since the beginning of recorded history. The serpent adopted as a logotype by the Institute of Medicine is a relief carving from ancient Greece, now held by the Staatliche Museen in Berlin.

Suggested citation: IOM (Institute of Medicine). 2015. *Enabling rapid and sustainable public health research during disasters: Summary of a joint workshop.* Washington, DC: The National Academies Press.

"Knowing is not enough; we must apply.
Willing is not enough; we must do."

—Goethe

INSTITUTE OF MEDICINE

OF THE NATIONAL ACADEMIES

Advising the Nation. Improving Health.

THE NATIONAL ACADEMIES

Advisers to the Nation on Science, Engineering, and Medicine

The **National Academy of Sciences** is a private, nonprofit, self-perpetuating society of distinguished scholars engaged in scientific and engineering research, dedicated to the furtherance of science and technology and to their use for the general welfare. Upon the authority of the charter granted to it by the Congress in 1863, the Academy has a mandate that requires it to advise the federal government on scientific and technical matters. Dr. Ralph J. Cicerone is president of the National Academy of Sciences.

The **National Academy of Engineering** was established in 1964, under the charter of the National Academy of Sciences, as a parallel organization of outstanding engineers. It is autonomous in its administration and in the selection of its members, sharing with the National Academy of Sciences the responsibility for advising the federal government. The National Academy of Engineering also sponsors engineering programs aimed at meeting national needs, encourages education and research, and recognizes the superior achievements of engineers. Dr. C. D. Mote, Jr., is president of the National Academy of Engineering.

The **Institute of Medicine** was established in 1970 by the National Academy of Sciences to secure the services of eminent members of appropriate professions in the examination of policy matters pertaining to the health of the public. The Institute acts under the responsibility given to the National Academy of Sciences by its congressional charter to be an adviser to the federal government and, upon its own initiative, to identify issues of medical care, research, and education. Dr. Victor J. Dzau is president of the Institute of Medicine.

The **National Research Council** was organized by the National Academy of Sciences in 1916 to associate the broad community of science and technology with the Academy's purposes of furthering knowledge and advising the federal government. Functioning in accordance with general policies determined by the Academy, the Council has become the principal operating agency of both the National Academy of Sciences and the National Academy of Engineering in providing services to the government, the public, and the scientific and engineering communities. The Council is administered jointly by both Academies and the Institute of Medicine. Dr. Ralph J. Cicerone and Dr. C. D. Mote, Jr., are chair and vice chair, respectively, of the National Research Council.

www.national-academies.org

WORKSHOP PLANNING COMMITTEE[1]

DAVID ABRAMSON, National Center for Disaster Preparedness, Columbia University, New York, NY
GEORGES BENJAMIN, American Public Health Association, Washington, DC
BERNARD D. GOLDSTEIN, Department of Environmental and Occupational Health, University of Pittsburgh Graduate School of Public Health, PA
JACK HERRMANN, National Association of County and City Health Officials, Washington, DC
DAVID LAKEY, Texas Department of State Health Services, Austin
ROBERT J. URSANO, Department of Psychiatry, Uniformed Services University of the Health Sciences, Bethesda, MD
BEVERLY L. WRIGHT, Dillard University, New Orleans, LA
HOWARD ZUCKER, New York State Department of Health, New York

HHS Staff

STACEY ARNESEN, National Library of Medicine, National Institutes of Health
DIANE DIEULIIS, Office of the Assistant Secretary for Preparedness and Response
SAMUEL L. GROSECLOSE, Centers for Disease Control and Prevention
JOSEPH "CHIP" HUGHES, National Institute of Environmental Health Sciences, National Institutes of Health
AUBREY MILLER, National Institute of Environmental Health Sciences, National Institutes of Health

IOM Staff

BRUCE M. ALTEVOGT, Forum Director
MEGAN REEVE, Associate Program Officer
BRADLEY ECKERT, Research Associate (*until September 2014*)

---

[1]Institute of Medicine planning committees are solely responsible for organizing the workshop, identifying topics, and choosing speakers. The responsibility for the published workshop summary rests with the workshop rapporteurs and the institution.

ASHLEY OTTEWELL, Research Associate (*since September 2014*)
ALEX REPACE, Senior Program Assistant
ANDREW M. POPE, Director, Board on Health Sciences Policy

FORUM ON MEDICAL AND PUBLIC HEALTH PREPAREDNESS FOR CATASTROPHIC EVENTS[1]

[1]Institute of Medicine forums and roundtables do not issue, review, or approve individual documents. The responsibility for the published workshop summary rests with the workshop rapporteurs and the institution.

LISA G. KAPLOWITZ, Office of the Assistant Secretary for Preparedness and Response, Department of Health and Human Services, Washington, DC
ALI S. KHAN, Centers for Disease Control and Prevention, Atlanta, GA (*until September 2014*)
MICHAEL G. KURILLA, National Institute of Allergy and Infectious Diseases, Washington, DC
DONALD M. LUMPKINS, Federal Emergency Management Agency, Department of Homeland Security, Washington, DC (*since March 2014*)
JAYNE LUX, National Business Group on Health, Washington, DC
LINDA M. MacINTYRE, American Red Cross, San Rafael, CA
SUZET M. McKINNEY, Chicago Department of Public Health, Chicago, IL
NICOLE McKOIN, Target Corporation, Furlong, PA
MARGARET M. McMAHON, Emergency Nurses Association, Williamstown, NJ (*until January 2014*)
AUBREY K. MILLER, National Institute of Environmental Health Sciences, Bethesda, MD
MATTHEW MINSON, Texas A&M University, College Station
ERIN MULLEN, Pharmaceutical Research and Manufacturers of America, Washington, DC
JOHN OSBORN, Mayo Clinic, Rochester, MN
ANDREW T. PAVIA, Infectious Disease Society of America, Salt Lake City, UT
STEVEN J. PHILLIPS, National Library of Medicine, Bethesda, MD
LEWIS J. RADONOVICH, Department of Veterans Affairs, Washington, DC
SONIA A. RASMUSSEN, Centers for Disease Control and Prevention, Atlanta, GA (*since September 2014*)
MARY J. RILEY, Administration for Children and Families, Department of Health and Human Services, Washington, DC
KENNETH W. SCHOR, Uniformed Services University of the Health Sciences, Bethesda, MD
ROSLYNE SCHULMAN, American Hospital Association, Washington, DC
RICHARD SERINO, Harvard School of Public Health, Boston, MA
MARGARET VANAMRINGE, The Joint Commission, Washington, DC

W. CRAIG VANDERWAGEN, Martin, Blanck & Associates, Alexandria, VA
JENNIFER WARD, Trauma Center Association of America, Las Cruces, NM
JOHN M. WIESMAN, Washington State Department of Health, Tumwater
GAMUNU WIJETUNGE, National Highway Traffic Safety Administration, Washington, DC

IOM Staff

BRUCE M. ALTEVOGT, Forum Director
MEGAN REEVE, Associate Program Officer
BRADLEY ECKERT, Research Associate (*until September 2014*)
ASHLEY OTTEWELL, Research Associate (*since September 2014*)
ALEX REPACE, Senior Program Assistant
ANDREW M. POPE, Director, Board on Health Sciences Policy

Reviewers

This workshop summary has been reviewed in draft form by individuals chosen for their diverse perspectives and technical expertise, in accordance with procedures approved by the National Research Council's Report Review Committee. The purpose of this independent review is to provide candid and critical comments that will assist the institution in making its published workshop summary as sound as possible and to ensure that the workshop summary meets institutional standards for objectivity, evidence, and responsiveness to the study charge. The review comments and draft manuscript remain confidential to protect the integrity of the process. We wish to thank the following individuals for their review of this workshop summary:

NELL ALLBRITTON, Louisiana Department of Health and Hospitals
J. PERREN COBB, Massachusetts General Hospital
SALLY PHILLIPS, Department of Homeland Security
ALONZO PLOUGH, Robert Wood Johnson Foundation

Although the reviewers listed above have provided many constructive comments and suggestions, they did not see the final draft of the workshop summary before its release. The review of this workshop summary was overseen by **KRISTINE GEBBIE,** Flinders University School of Nursing and Midwifery. Appointed by the Institute of Medicine, she was responsible for making certain that an independent examination of this workshop summary was carried out in accordance with institutional procedures and that all review comments were carefully considered. Responsibility for the final content of this workshop summary rests entirely with the rapporteurs and the institution.

Contents

1

Introduction[1]

Over the past decade, preparedness and response capacities of government agencies, hospitals and clinics, public health agencies, and academic researchers in the United States and abroad have been challenged by a succession of public health emergencies, ranging from radiological threats to pandemics to earthquakes. Through After Action Reports, each of these emergencies has yielded important information and lessons learned that can inform future disaster response and recovery efforts. However, important information that needs to be collected during and immediately following these emergencies is often missed because of barriers and obstacles to gathering such data, such as varying institutional review board (IRB) restrictions in different states, no sustainable funding network for this type of work, uncertainty on who should be involved in research response, and a lack of knowledge around how best to integrate research into response and recovery frameworks. Another challenge, said Aubrey Miller, senior medical adviser at the National Institute of Environmental Health Sciences (NIEHS), is how to enable science faster during a disaster to address the important health questions more quickly. Nicole Lurie, Assistant Secretary for Preparedness and Response, observed that although issues and challenges have been discussed for years in numerous different venues, there is now a groundswell of interest across all sectors in moving beyond discussion

[1]The planning committee's role was limited to planning the workshop. This workshop summary has been prepared by the rapporteurs as a factual summary of what occurred at the workshop. Statements, recommendations, and opinions expressed are those of individual presenters and participants, and are not necessarily endorsed or verified by the Institute of Medicine and should not be construed as reflecting any group consensus.

and taking action. Public health and other local agencies around the country have many ongoing community resilience and preparedness activities, so building disaster research efforts by integrating into already established frameworks could prevent duplication and augment funding support. She encouraged working to operationalize these issues in science preparedness and response and highlighted integrating research framework into existing response frame-works, implementing plans that support research into real-world responses, and building new relationships between research networks and the responding community.

Taking action to enable medical and public health research during disasters was the focus of a workshop held on June 12 and 13, 2014, on the campus of the National Institutes of Health (NIH) in Bethesda, Maryland. It was coordinated and supported jointly by the Institute of Medicine (IOM) Forum on Medical and Public Health Preparedness for Catastrophic Events, NIEHS, the National Library of Medicine (NLM), the U.S. Department of Health and Human Services' (HHS's) Office of the Assistant Secretary for Preparedness and Response (ASPR), and the U.S. Centers for Disease Control and Prevention (CDC). Invited speakers and participants from federal, state, and local government, academia, and community and worker organizations came together to discuss how to integrate research into existing response structures; identify critical research needs and priorities; identify obstacles and barriers to research; discuss structures and strategies needed for deployment of a research study; share ideas, innovations, and technologies to support research; and explore data collection tools and data-sharing mechanisms for both rapid and longitudinal research.

Lurie and Miller challenged participants to outline the top action items for improving national and local capabilities to enhance medium to longer-term health research. Specifically, they asked participants to consider: Which individuals would perform research (and what is the role of citizen science)? What logistical support, training, or protocols are needed to collect data in the field? How should the data be managed, and what are the ethical and legal concerns? How should risk communication be facilitated among researchers, health officials, and the community? Who else needs to be involved in the research proposals and data collection (and what is the role of private industry, workers, others)? The objectives for the workshop discussions as outlined by the workshop planning committee are presented in Box 1-1.[2]

---

[2]The full Statement of Task can be found in Appendix F.

BOX 1-1
Workshop Objectives

The workshop will examine strategies and diversified partnerships to enable methodologically and ethically sound public health and medical research during future emergencies. Specific goals include discussions of

- Ensuring adequate protections for human research participants, including informed consent during emergencies.
- Issues and new efforts in development to enable institutions to use central Institutional Review Boards for public health emergencies.
- Strategies and resources to help support timely research by investigators and research institutions while reducing deployment times and administrative burden.
    - Decision-making triggers to activate identified research efforts.
    - Important infrastructure gaps and short-term opportunities to advance research responses.
- Effective integration and implementation of research efforts alongside life-saving emergency response activities and platforms (e.g., logistics, communications, access, safety).
    - Opportunities and challenges associated with establishing "researcher response" teams.
- Improved involvement and coordination among government, academia, and the community to facilitate needed research infrastructure and timely responses, including use of "citizen science," into a research response framework.

ORGANIZATION OF THE WORKSHOP AND REPORT

In addition to several overview presentations and case examples, the workshop was organized around focused panel discussions on six key areas identified by the workshop planning committee as relevant to advancing research response capabilities (see Box 1-2).

The following report summarizes the presentations from expert speakers and discussions among workshop participants. Chapter 2 provides a brief background on conducting research during disasters, including several current federal disaster research initiatives and resources. Chapter 3 presents some lessons learned from recent disasters

BOX 1-2
Six Key Topic Areas

1. Addressing institutional review board barriers to health research implementation.
2. Partnering with the community to enable access and baseline data.
3. Improving data collection capabilities and information resources.
4. Considerations for rapid and sustained funding mechanisms for research in disasters.
5. Improving the role of extramural clinical and academic researchers, centers, and networks.
6. Coordinating logistics to execute rapid research in disaster response.

regarding medical and public health research needs and actions. Cases explored include Hurricanes Katrina and Sandy, the Deepwater Horizon oil spill, and the 9/11 terrorist attacks. Chapters 4 through 9 include overviews of the six breakout panel sessions, including the facilitators' reports on the key issues and opportunities highlighted by participants in each session. Finally, Chapter 10 summarizes the reflections of the response panel and their comments on taking the field of disaster research forward.

OVERVIEW OF TOPICS HIGHLIGHTED DURING PRESENTATIONS AND DISCUSSIONS[3]

A number of themes emerged across multiple workshop presentations and discussions as participants considered potential opportunities for improving research in disaster response across the six focus areas listed. The themes and opportunities highlighted below (see Box 1-3), as identified by one or more individual participants are, expanded upon below the box as in succeeding chapters.

[3]Rapporteurs' summary of main topics and recurring themes from the presentations, discussions, and summary remarks by the meeting and session chairs. Items on this list should not be construed as reflecting any consensus of the workshop participants or any endorsement by the IOM or the Forum.

BOX 1-3
Themes and Opportunities During Workshop Discussions

- Actionable science, with the ultimate goal of improving outcomes for those impacted by disaster
- Defining the key questions
- Defining the "research responders"
- Rapid and agile funding mechanisms
- Core dataset
    - Standardization
    - Building day-to-day systems, networks, and trust
- Streamline IRB approval process
- Coordination of research across studies and into the larger emergency management system
- Essential partnerships
    - The community
    - Public health agencies and the health care sector
    - Local academic institutions
    - Unions, workers' organizations, and workers
    - Disaster epidemiologists
    - Emergency medical services (EMS)
    - Pharmaceutical manufacturers and pharmacists
    - Funding partners

- **Actionable science, with the ultimate goal of improving outcomes for those impacted by disaster.** A main theme underpinning all discussions was the need for timely collection of data during disasters to improve science preparedness and medical and public health response efforts (not simply collecting data). Many participants stressed that any research conducted during a disaster should be relevant and meaningful, with the goal of enhancing response and improving human health outcomes.
- **Defining the key questions.** Honing the actionable medical and public health science theme further, many participants highlighted the benefit to clearly define the questions to be answered by research during a disaster.
- **Defining the "research responders."** Having pre-identified networks and rosters of responders with specific types of expertise that can be matched to the disaster needs would aid in

creating a more efficient study process. Some participants suggested having a cadre of volunteers and professionals on reserve, similar to the Medical Reserve Corps volunteers, who are trained in the response structure of disasters but also have identified and documented skills that can be used when needed. Technology and increased crowdsourcing opportunities also create the prospect for "citizen scientists" and engaging people at the community level who know baseline information, understand the cultural nuances, and will be invested in the outcomes of the science response.

- **Rapid and agile funding mechanisms.** Having nimble funding opportunities that can be flexible to situational needs and quick to deploy is an ongoing challenge. Academic institutions and government have difficulty holding onto nondescript funding that may not be used each fiscal year. Some models discussed could serve as potential methods, such as the National Science Foundation's (NSF's) RAPID model and the Natural Hazards Center in Colorado. Making the case that disaster research can be directly linked to impact disaster response decisions and community resiliency can also help to include research in more routine disaster funding.
- **Core dataset.** Much of the discussion was focused on the challenges of determining the core set of data elements that need to be collected once key questions are identified. Data collection, in particular, has been an ongoing challenge, including the ability to deploy rapidly and immediately begin to collect what was referred to as perishable or ephemeral baseline data.

    - **Standardization.** Participants discussed the need for a standardized, minimum set of data elements that would be sought by anyone collecting data. Participants also discussed the need for common terminology and definitions and the development of standardized data collection and reporting tools. A centralized list (website) of tools and disaster literature was also suggested.
    - **Building day-to-day systems, networks, and trust.** Various participants advocated for building strong health care infrastructure and systems that can provide care to everyone on a day-to-day basis, rather than developing separate systems to be used only in a disaster. This way,

systems that already collect data on a routine basis can be tapped easily for research needs in a disaster. Data collection functions could even be integrated into existing incident command system frameworks to ensure continuity. There was also much emphasis on establishing strong predisaster networks, coalitions, and trust relationships that can be rapidly accessed during a disaster when the need for data arises. Some participants also discussed systemic rostering of people in these networks—assembling lists of experts so that teams can be more easily and rapidly assembled after a disaster.

- **Streamline IRB approval process.** Participants discussed issues of IRB approval, the value and role of a central or national rapid IRB for use in disasters (e.g., the Public Health Emergency Research Review Board, or PHERRB), and the possibility of preapproval of protocols and methodology to expedite study deployment. With regard to informed consent, several participants raised the issue of therapeutic misconception and highlighted the need to ensure that potential participants fully understand the difference between research and services before participating, especially during a crisis when they are most vulnerable.
- **Coordination of research across studies and into the larger emergency management system.** Several participants highlighted the advantages of coordination among institutions, IRBs, and the federal entities funding the research. The potential for "survey fatigue" among research participants was noted, given the large number of research projects being done concurrently in a disaster. There were also calls for coordination of research with the incident command structure (ICS) and defining where research fits within the emergency management structure.
- **Essential partnerships.** Another recurring discussion point was that no single researcher, team, discipline, agency, or institution alone can address these issues. Leveraging the strengths of many different partners is necessary, including funding partners to make this research truly multidisciplinary. A few participants pointed out, however, that academic institutions are not funded for relationship building and highlighted challenges of establishing and funding a sustainable ready reserve base. Essential partners listed by participants included

- **The community,** as both participants in research and partners in collecting data. Community members and leaders have many resources that can be brought to bear, including their networks and their experience with, for example, advocacy, community meetings, and mobilizations. The community has a wealth of knowledge regarding how they, as a community, can best be engaged and what best serves their needs in their environment. Several participants supported the idea of having an ongoing relationship of trust with the community, sharing findings and helping them to understand the value of research. Some participants also discussed engaging the community in data collection efforts and fostering "citizen science."
- **Public health agencies and the health care sector** can both inform key research questions and help to apply the information gleaned in a practical environment while also acting as data sources for various types of studies. Additionally, to support the suggestions to make better connections with the community, public health and health care can encourage access to affected persons/populations to capture essential information to support research efforts during response.
- **Local academic institutions,** who have a vested interest in the community and who can help to provide baseline data, conduct studies, facilitate stakeholder meetings, provide surge capacity (e.g., staff, space for shelters), assess training needs, provide technical assistance, and collaborate on publications.
- **Unions, workers' organizations, and workers,** including employees of impacted companies/facilities as well as a broad range of emergency responders; public health, medical and social workers; skilled support workers; workers involved in the cleanup; construction labor; and others.
- **Disaster epidemiologists,** as providers of baseline data. As a partner discipline, disaster epidemiology can offer rapid needs assessments, shelter surveillance, morbidity and mortality surveillance, responder health and safety surveillance, descriptive and analytic studies, evaluation and impact studies, and registries.
- **Emergency medical services,** as a valuable source of data during and after disasters. The National EMS Information

System (NEMSIS) could potentially provide baseline information, the capacity to conduct longitudinal health assessments for high-risk groups, and deidentified data.

- **Pharmaceutical manufacturers and pharmacists,** who have a lot of information about their products that may not be in the public domain. They could, for example, assist with the development of postevent study protocols involving their products, contribute unique analytic capabilities, have a role in the conduct and analysis of studies, and develop patient communications.
- **Funding partners,** including federal funders, health foundations, corporate donors, and others. It was noted that private foundations generally move much faster than the typical government agency and have a strong community-orientation focus. Participants discussed that funding is needed not only for the study of the clinical and technological aspects of response, but also for the study of organizational management (e.g., coordination, communication, situational assessment, and data sharing). Funding is also needed before events to develop infrastructure and instruments and to be ready to arrive at the site as soon as possible and characterize the exposures by whatever means are appropriate before ephemeral data dissipate.

2

Science Preparedness: Conducting Research During Public Health Emergencies

The H1N1 influenza pandemic in 2009 highlighted the challenges of doing scientific research in the face of a public health crisis, said Assistant Secretary for Preparedness and Response Nicole Lurie in her keynote address. She highlighted several successes, such as the rapid characterization of the virus, determining the vaccine dose for children, surveillance for antigenic drift, and standardized data collection using existing adult and pediatric critical care research networks. However, there were also real shortcomings, for example, delays in human subjects review that limited real-time data sharing and analysis, important research questions that were not considered until it was too late to act on them, and limited biospecimen collection. Other disasters in years following 2009 also illustrated the need for a robust science response, and multiple federal agencies have begun partnering on projects to accomplish this in a coordinated and streamlined manner.

CHALLENGES AND GAPS

Lurie also shared her personal experience with the challenges of data sharing and research during H1N1 and other disasters. After speaking with intensive care physicians, Lurie sought to collect data to develop practice guidelines for managing critical patients with H1N1 influenza. She approached the Acute Respiratory Distress Syndrome Research Network (ARDSNet), which had an organized research network and was able to rapidly modify its data collection protocol to gather data during the pandemic. Unfortunately, no data were submitted, as participating institutions had to get IRB approval to change their protocols to be able to submit deidentified data, a process that took up to 6 months. Eighteen months later it was learned that 40 percent of the children who died succumbed to resistant *Staphylococcus* infections, not H1N1—critical information that could have guided practice had it been known in a timely fashion.

Many similar research challenges were present in subsequent disasters. For example, real-time collection and analysis of data during the January 2010 earthquake in Haiti would have allowed for development of more granular clinical guidelines on treating complex fractures in austere environments, Lurie said. Following the Deepwater Horizon oil spill in the Gulf of Mexico in April 2010, the IOM convened a science workshop in the Gulf at the request of HHS to consider how to assess the effects of the spill on human health[1] (IOM, 2010). At that workshop it was discussed that despite nearly 40 major oil spills in the past 50 years, all involving some kind of oil and some kind of dispersant, data remain very limited on the impacts of oil and dispersants on health. Each of those oil spills also had important behavioral health sequelae, yet there was little information on preventive behavioral health interventions. During the 2011 Japan nuclear disaster, it became clear that the United States has a limited number of experts in radiation exposure, limited laboratory capacity to handle radiation disasters, and inconsistent guidance on the use of potassium iodide.

BUILDING A ROBUST SCIENCE RESPONSE

Together, the after-action reports for each of these events demonstrate the need to do a better job of "scientific research in response," Lurie said. This means strengthening the evidence base to inform preparedness and making decisions with the best available science. In this regard, the process for expert analysis and advice should be formally integrated into the command structure for response, she said. A process is also needed that links that best available science with research needs, a process to rapidly prioritize gaps and execute the research to resolve critical questions before the next disaster event.

To begin to address these gaps, Lurie and colleagues from NIH and CDC set out to define the basic components required to build a robust

---

[1]Additional information on this workshop can be found at http://iom.edu/Reports/2010/Research-Priorities-for-Assessing-Health-Effects-from-the-Gulf-of-Mexico-Oil-Spill.aspx (accessed September 14, 2014).

science response and what would be needed to make them operational (see Table 2-1), publishing an article in the *New England Journal of Medicine*. Lawrence Taybak, principal deputy director of NIH, quoted from the article that "public health emergencies, especially those that result from natural disasters, are inevitable. The failure to use research to improve our response to future disasters is not" (Lurie et al., 2013, p. 1255). Tayback added that Francis Collins, director of NIH and an author on the paper, has stressed the urgent need to develop a multifaceted plan that allows for a swift and flexible response to disasters of the future. Lurie highlighted progress in implementing some of the components, including the development of rosters of experts for some threat areas and a pilot of the process for rapid identification of research priorities during the emergence of Middle East respiratory syndrome coronavirus (MERS-CoV).

The expertise for a robust science response exists, but bureaucratic, logistical, and financial obstacles can impede strategic science. NIH has

TABLE 2-1 Components of a Robust Science Response

Components	Making It Operational
Rostered experts in research design, technology, and topical areas of concern	Identify and roster experts; plan for "ready reserve" of citizen scientists and clinicians
Scientific research is part of core response plans	Make formal part of planning documents and incident command structure
Identification of knowledge gaps and research questions	Explicitly review, prioritize, and recommend which research to pursue
Generic and scenario-specific templates and protocols	Preapproved core survey documents; prescripted clinical protocols; minimum dataset
Rapid-review mechanisms for human subjects research	Advance approval, national review board for emergencies
Rapid funding	Implement administrative mechanisms to enable
Registries and networks for studies	Preprepared registries

Components	Making It Operational
Involvement of affected communities	Establish mechanisms to directly engage community to discuss concerns; share findings

SOURCE: Lurie presentation, June 12, 2014, adapted from Lurie et al. (2013).

been working on several pilot policies to enable scientific research in response. For example, the United States has more than 138 clinical research networks. With the appropriate level of guidance and infrastructure support, Lurie said, some of these networks could be used to support collaborative medical and public health research during an emergency. The PHERRB is another mechanism that NIH is developing. It is a rapid, centralized IRB, an intramural entity positioned to review protocols quickly during an emergency. NIH is working with 20 select institutions in these clinical networks to develop "reliance agreements," a legal agreement under which the institution agrees to rely on the PHERRB in an emergency. Lurie also suggested that the terms and conditions of awards could be used to facilitate rapid research. If a research network receives federal funding, it could, for example, be required to commit to the IRB review within 72 hours in the event of a disaster. Another policy approach is to expand access of the research community to datasets after an emergency event. For example, de-identified data from the Centers for Medicare & Medicaid Services (CMS) claims could be linked with data from the Federal Emergency Management Agency (FEMA) about who received what kind of assistance, or with data from the Department of Housing and Urban Development about housing, Census data, or other data to enable research.

Lurie described a pilot of the process to identify a research agenda, secure rapid funding, and work collaboratively to initiate the research. Following Hurricane Sandy in 2012, HHS asked the IOM and the New York Academy of Medicine (NYAM) to convene stakeholders in New York to define priority areas for recovery research less than 2 weeks after the storm.[2] Participants helped identify priorities in health system response research, community resilience, mold mitigation and related health issues, morbidity and mortality among at-risk and general populations, workforce health and response, evacuation and policy decision making and health outcomes, and mental health outcomes.

[2]Additional information on the NYAM meeting can be found at http://www.nyam.org/news/docs/pdf/NYAM-Disaster-Research-Priorities-Meeting-Summary.pdf (accessed October 13, 2014).

Funding was secured through the emergency supplemental appropriations for Sandy disaster relief,[3] and a collaborative effort among NIEHS, CDC, and ASPR awarded a series of grants for research in the identified priority areas (CDC, 2014). Although this was unique and fast moving for federal-level funding, grantees did not receive awards until 9 months after the hurricane, so there is still room for improvement.

Going forward, Lurie stressed the importance of continuing to build partnerships and relationships with local science research responders and clinical networks and to work toward prescripted clinical research protocols. To operationalize science preparedness and response efforts, she highlighted the need to; build research response into the incident command framework for disasters; test, train, and exercise plans (e.g., PHERRB); implement plans and policy tools that support research into real-world responses; develop and test tracking and exposure technologies; and develop and test capabilities for biospecimen collection.[4]

FEDERAL DISASTER RESEARCH INITIATIVES AND RESOURCES

As background for the panel discussions, speakers representing the federal sponsors of the workshop provided brief overviews of several current federal disaster research initiatives and resources, including the NIH Disaster Research Response Project, the National Institute for Occupational Safety and Health (NIOSH) Emergency Responder Health Monitoring and Surveillance System (ERHMS), the NIOSH Disaster Science Research Initiative, and the NLM Disaster Information Management Research Center.

NIH Disaster Research Response Project

As summarized by Linda Birnbaum, director of NIEHS and the National Toxicology Program, the main questions to be answered by research during and after a disaster are, What are the health implications of the exposures and stressors, both acute and long term, especially

---

[3]For the full text of the Disaster Relief Appropriations Act, see http://www.gpo.gov/fdsys/pkg/PLAW-113publ2/pdf/PLAW-113publ2.pdf (accessed September 9, 2014).

[4]For further information about the ASPR science preparedness initiative, see http://www.phe.gov/Preparedness/planning/science/Pages/default.aspx (accessed November 3, 2014).

among those who are most vulnerable (e.g., the young, old, sick, poor, disadvantaged)? Are the impacted areas safe places in which to live and work? What do we need to know to protect the public, both in the short and the long terms and to prepare for the future? One of the key challenges is getting information in a timely way.

Birnbaum introduced the NIH Disaster Research Response Project[5] (DR2), a pilot project initiated, in part, in direct response to the previously mentioned article by Lurie and colleagues in the *New England Journal of Medicine* (Lurie et al., 2013). The goal of the project, developed by NIEHS in collaboration with NLM, is to create a disaster research system consisting of research data collection tools and a network of trained research responders. NIEHS and NLM are developing a central repository for data collection tools and research protocols, available on the NLM Disaster Lit website.[6] NIEHS is developing an Intramural Fast Data Collection Team that is ready to mobilize in the event of a disaster to collect baseline, epidemiology, and clinical data, as well as biospecimens, using "plug and play" preexisting IRB-approved protocols. The NIEHS Worker Education and Training Program (WETP) is also working on developing training materials that can be used by NIH intramural and extramural researchers on how to safely conduct research in an emergency situation.

Birnbaum described a DR2 tabletop exercise held at the port of Los Angeles in April 2014, involving about 140 participants from federal, state, and local government; academia (NIEHS-funded centers and grantees); and community partners. The scenario was an earthquake-induced tsunami approaching the ports of Los Angeles and Long Beach, which are very industrialized areas with a large number of ships, tankers, oil storage areas, and train depots, as well as homes and schools. The exercise included a bus tour through the port, where it became clear that people who were in the port area when a tsunami hit could have great difficulty escaping. Participants then discussed how to incorporate health researchers into response and recovery efforts in the hypothetical disaster scenario, including barriers to data collection and ways to overcome them. Birnbaum showed a brief video of highlights from the exercise and referred participants to a report of the findings on the NIEHS website.[7]

---

[5]For more on this multiagency project, see http://sis.nlm.nih.gov/dimrc/dr2/disaster research. html (accessed on December 12, 2014).

[6]See http://disasterlit.nlm.nih.gov (accessed on December 12, 2014).

[7]The report and additional information about the exercise are available at http://tools.niehs.nih.gov/wetp/events.cfm?id=2537 (accessed December 12, 2014).

Looking forward, Birnbaum said there are opportunities to build on DR2 and other efforts, and she encouraged participants to look for opportunities for rapid collection of environmental data to go with health data and to continue to develop collaborations with federal, state, academic, and community partners, as well as industrial partners who have a great stake in the communities in which they are located. She also noted the need to explore the role of new technologies (e.g., mobile health, social media) and use the "citizen science" approach in research. NIEHS intends to hold future exercises to test the research response strategies and protocols being developed to be able to implement them in the field, and to continue to improve training.

NIOSH Emergency Responder Health Monitoring and Surveillance System

Based on experiences with a number of disasters—Hurricane Katrina in particular—NIOSH saw the need to develop a systematic approach to health monitoring and surveillance across all phases of responder involvement in a disaster (predeployment, deployment, and post-deployment). John Howard, director of NIOSH, explained that ERHMS was developed to provide tools and guidance focused on ensuring that only qualified, trained, and properly equipped personnel (employees, contractors, and volunteers) are selected for deployment and that all responders receive sufficient health and exposure monitoring. Activities addressed by ERHMS in each phase of deployment, as listed by Howard, are shown in Figure 2-1.[8] The ERHMS technical assistance document was approved by the National Response Team[9] for use by responders and those involved in the deployment of responders, including incident commanders, emergency managers, and agency heads.

---

[8]For further information on ERHMS, see http://www.cdc.gov/niosh/topics/erhms and http://nrt.sraprod.com/ERHMS (accessed October 9, 2014).

[9]The National Response Team is an organization of 15 federal departments and agencies responsible for coordinating preparedness and response to hazardous substance pollution incidents. See http://www.nrt.org (accessed November 10, 2014).

NIOSH Disaster Science Research Initiative

In January 2014, NIOSH launched the Disaster Science Research Initiative to develop a framework for an approach to timely, scalable, and scientifically sound research. The framework allows for research to be started quickly at the beginning, during, and after the response to a large-scale disaster. Areas of investigation include responder demographic ascertainment (i.e., rostering); exposure assessment (direct reading and sensor technology; real-time, continuous air monitoring; biomonitoring; analytics); personal protective equipment selection, use, and effectiveness; and responder mental health and resiliency. Responder resilience is the ability to rapidly adjust to adversity without physiological or psychological adverse effect, and is an integral component of health and safety (Reissman et al., 2009, 2011).

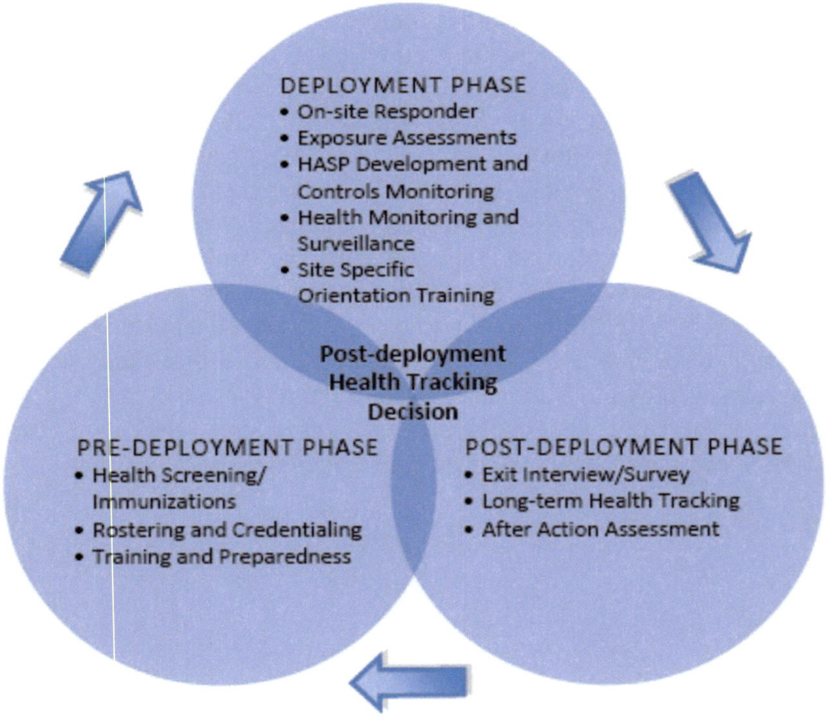

FIGURE 2-1 Emergency Responder Health Monitoring and Surveillance System comprehensive approach to responder health and safety.
NOTE: HASP = health and safety plan.
SOURCE: Howard presentation, June 12, 2014.

Howard noted that NIOSH has developed a number of direct reading instruments for workplace monitoring that have been patented and licensed. A well-known example is the personal dust monitor carried by coal miners. NIOSH is also studying biomarkers of exposure and the potential uses of in-dwelling monitors enabled by nanosensors that can send data to a central database (e.g., core temperature monitors in pill form). The goal is to make exposure detection faster so an individual can manipulate the environment and reduce exposure if necessary. Howard noted that determining when biological monitoring should be conducted can be difficult. For example, whether a scientific rationale exists for biological monitoring in a given situation, whether the monitoring results can provide meaningful and/or reliable information regarding health impact, or how such information would ultimately benefit the worker are questions to consider before implementing a monitoring system (Decker et al., 2013b).

Engaging Medical Librarians and the National Library of Medicine

Donald Lindberg, director of NLM, called attention to NLM's vast resources, including the Disaster Information Management Re-search Center, which houses extensive health information resources and technology for disaster preparedness, response, and recovery.[10] He urged participants to use these resources and those of medical libraries more generally. NLM and medical librarians should be included in planning for disaster management and recovery, he said. Specifically, he suggested that NLM could be called on to organize the published academic and noncommercial information relevant to disaster planning research and recovery for archiving and for immediate retrieval. He added that he would welcome an explicit request and the authority to organize the gray literature on disasters. Lindberg explained that many reports and resources are not as easily available as most would expect, and some can be very difficult to find, depending on how they are indexed or posted on the Internet. He also pointed out that there is an emerging specialist group of medical librarians called Disaster Information Specialists; these informaticians can be embedded in NIH research grants and paid for by NLM.

[10]See http://disasterinfo.nlm.nih.gov (accessed November 3, 2014).

3

Health Research Needs and Actions: Lessons from Recent Disasters

A succession of public health emergencies and disasters in the past decade has challenged capacities both in the United States and abroad (Lurie et al., 2013). Each one is unique, but there are generalizable elements and common barriers and facilitators to response that can be learned from them. Bob Ursano, chair of the Department of Psychiatry and Director of the Center for the Study of Traumatic Stress at the Uniformed Services University of the Health Sciences, reiterated Lurie's comments regarding the need to produce actionable science—not just research, but science preparedness and response. What are the research questions of most importance, what are the targets for answering those questions, what are the tools for accomplishing the research, and what are the resources that can be brought to bear and impediments to be overcome? This chapter considers the lessons learned from recent disasters regarding health research needs and actions, including examples of strong cohort participation and elements to support rapid funding. Cases explored include the 9/11 terrorist attacks, Hurricane Katrina in 2005, the Deepwater Horizon oil spill in 2010, and Hurricane Sandy in 2012.

SEPTEMBER 11, 2001

Because disasters are unexpected, disaster research is inherently different from nondisaster research. In nondisaster research, scientists plan, collect data, analyze that data, and develop an intervention. In a disaster, intervention (i.e., the response to the disaster) must be immediate. Data collection occurs under difficult circumstances and is confounded by the ongoing interventions and other stressors. Analysis of data is also impacted. David Prezant, chief medical officer for the Fire Department of New York City (FDNY), shared his perspectives on research challenges and lessons learned based on his experiences during the World Trade Center (WTC) rescue and recovery efforts following the terrorist attacks of September 11, 2001.

Why Research During a Response

Because funding and staffing situations can be fragile, questions on the need for research or activities not directly related to an emergency response are perpetually raised. Prezant elucidated an important example showing the need for timely research specifically related to the disaster at hand. As a result of the 2001 attacks in New York, two 110-story towers and several surrounding buildings were reduced to about four stories of pulverized rubble. What was not in the rubble pile was suspended in the air in an enormous dust cloud. Shortly after the collapse of the towers, news outlets were interviewing experts on television, some of whom said there would be no respiratory effects of exposure to the debris dust cloud. They based these statements, Prezant explained, on research that has demonstrated that particles must be less than 3 microns in size to enter the lower airways. At the very most, they predicted mild upper airway consequences (chronic sinusitis, rhinitis). These experts were wrong, Prezant said, because they were thinking about low-density, low-concentration inhalation experiments as would occur with tuberculosis or other infection agents or with metered-dose inhalers. This exposure lasted for several days, and about 16,000 FDNY rescue workers continued to be exposed to different levels of dust in encapsulated sub-terranean areas over the next 10 months during the intense rescue and recovery effort.

Prezant said firefighters came out of the rubble and told him that the air had a different smell and taste than anything they had experienced before in fighting fires. The firefighters at the WTC site were exposed to high concentrations of very alkaline dust (approximate pH of 10) containing a mixture of pulverized cement, gypsum, pulverized glass, asbestos, silica, fibrous glass, heavy metals, volatile organic compounds, and the organic combustion/pyrolysis products of all the building components and jet fuel (e.g., polycyclic aromatic hydrocarbons, dioxins, polychlorinated biphenyls). About 3 weeks into the recovery effort, a therapeutic, diagnostic bronchoscopic evaluation of a firefighter who was sent to a nearby hospital in respiratory distress and arrest revealed uncoated asbestos fibers, glass, and pulverized ash. In other cases, macrophages in sputum samples collected 10 months after 9/11 contained encapsulated dust similar to that at the WTC site (Fireman et al., 2004). Air and respiratory monitoring while the response and clean-up was going on might have allowed responders and clinicians to more quickly see the potential hazards involved and change actions accordingly.

The Importance of Early Baseline Data

In many disasters, baseline data may not exist or are hard to access for the same cohort looking to be studied. This lack of access can make it even more difficult to pinpoint causes or link health outcomes to disaster exposures. Prezant also stressed the importance of acting immediately to get monitoring and treatment systems in place, so that data are not lost and so that credibility as a partner is established. An FDNY WTC responder cohort was established after 9/11, and a well-organized medical monitoring program has minimized longitudinal dropout with consistently high retention rates (92–95 percent). Because FDNY has been capturing health data, including pulmonary function tests, systematically since 1996, this is the only cohort with pre-9/11 health data, Prezant noted. This cohort also has the highest exposure to respiratory irritants and combustion by-products of any WTC cohort. Monitoring and treatment protocols are in place for respiratory and mental health issues as well as for late emerging diseases (e.g., cancer). This can also foster trust with participants by allowing them to be cared for quickly, which will continue to encourage study involvement and high retention (see Figure 3-1).

Coordinating Logistics to Execute Rapid and Sustained Research in Disaster Response

Research is a slow, deliberative, thoughtful, and collaborative process. Disaster research, however, has to absorb the immediacy of the event, Prezant said. Without that information, any of the outcomes of interest will remain elusive, regardless of the techniques used. The immediate data are essential to determine what did or did not happen; who was exposed, to what, and to what extent; and what the immediate

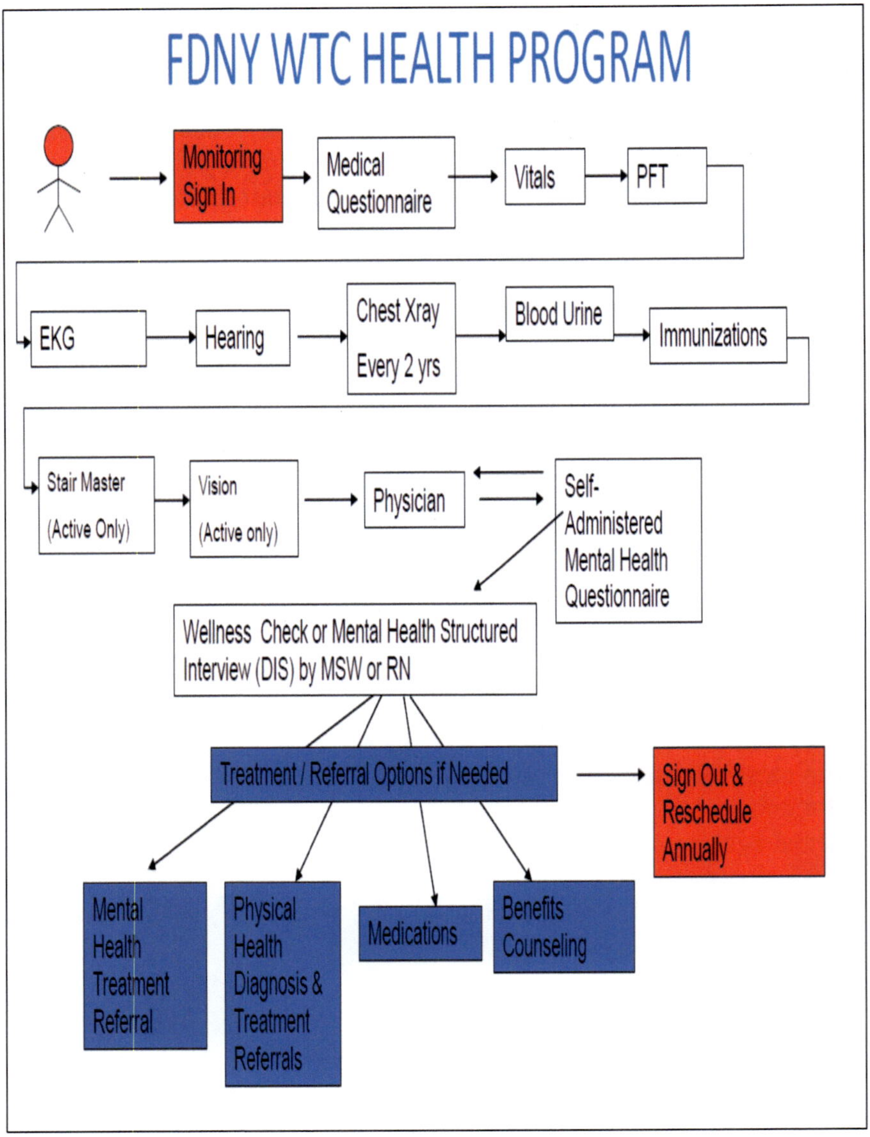

FIGURE 3-1 The World Trade Center Health Program for the Fire Department of New York.
NOTE: DIS = Diagnostic Interview Schedule; EKG = electrocardiogram; MSW = master of social work; PFT = Physical Fitness Test; RN = registered nurse.
SOURCE: Prezant presentation, June 12, 2014.

impact appears to be. The research questions are similar at every disaster, and preparedness requires prearranged studies that are ready to go, he added.

Partnering with Communities to Facilitate Pre-Event Assessment

Partnering with communities, Prezant said, including state and local government, is essential to facilitate access to pre-event data, collection of baseline data, and longitudinal assessment of the population (discussed further in Chapter 5). Participants need a reason to participate in research, Prezant continued; too often, participants view research as an experiment. They have already lived through one experiment (the disaster), and they are not inspired to volunteer for another. In addition, they are dealing with the aftermath of the disaster (e.g., the death of a loved one, loss of their home), and their energy and patience are limited. Therefore, participants need a reason to believe the research effort is worth their remaining energies and time. This involves developing trust, which requires credibility. IRB approval is not enough to garner trust and demonstrate credibility to people, Prezant said. They do not know what an IRB is. What is needed are partnerships and a history of service that preferably began before the disaster (as is seen with the FDNY responder cohort). There also needs to be a "stamp of excellence" from a major organization that the community trusts (e.g., the American Cancer Society, the American Heart Association, CDC) to help secure local buy-in and public labor and management support.

> Participation is maximized if everyone agrees that disaster research is not an experiment. It's a promise, with an end toward recovery.
> —*David Prezant*

If we cannot monitor, assess, provide services, intervene, and reassess, we cannot provide what people need in a disaster, Prezant said. If we do not know what is going on in the communities, we cannot respond, or we respond with the wrong interventions, only making matters worse, he continued. The end point then is not the data, but the knowledge that can be used to guide recovery, including clinical services and systems improvements. Continued participation requires fulfillment of this promise, in the form of delivery on end points in the short term as well as in the longer term.

As an example of delivering on the promise of research, Prezant cited several published papers on declining pulmonary function in WTC responders in the short term and persistence of reduced function in the long term (Aldrich et al., 2010; Banauch et al., 2006; Prezant et al., 2002). FDNY was also the first to publish an early assessment of cancer outcomes, showing a cancer signal only 7 years after 9/11. This affected federal health care policy, Prezant said, because cancer was then added to WTC covered conditions (Zeig-Owens et al., 2011).

FDNY is also involved in basic research. For example, blood banked during the first 6 months after 9/11 has been used for studies linking pulmonary function test outcomes to biomarkers that could potentially predict both susceptibility and resistance to disease (Cho et al., 2013; Nolan et al., 2012). Firefighters are saying yes to participating in basic science research, as long as they have a sense that it is going to help them or another firefighter who is exposed.

Obtaining Rapid and Sustained Research Funding

Research funding after a disaster has several phases, and they are generally based on public perception, Prezant said. Initially, small amounts of funding flow from governments and philanthropies because it is "the right thing to do." This is often followed by disbelief about whether people were actually exposed to something dangerous, whether it was just an acute issue that will resolve spontaneously, or whether the exposure actually caused disease. The next phase is apathy, when funders question whether this research is still important and how much is enough, especially in the face of other national priorities.

The way to overcome these barriers to funding is data-driven advocacy, which requires research, Prezant said. Emotional advocacy secures the initial funding to look at uncertain exposures or health effects, but without data to show importance, there is a loss of credibility. No study is ever perfect, and this is especially true for disaster research where there are numerous, simultaneous, and often unknown confounders. However, multiple studies showing similar effects lead to a more perfect understanding and a more perfect response (i.e., improved services and systems). Research requires educating everyone involved (researchers, participants, funding agencies) as to what is achievable given the situation and adjustment of expectations across all of the funding agencies.

Improving Research Systems and Data Collection

Although everyone thinks their idea is worthy of immediate study, and there are novel issues that can occur, we need to remain focused on the main questions, Prezant said. Affected systems and populations have limited time for testing and questionnaires, and overburdening people can lead to longitudinal dropout. In addition, trying to capture too much data can reduce focus and lead to paralysis. The questions, data collection, and analyses need to be part of a predisaster, agreed-upon, focused agenda, he said.

Data collection should allow for immediate collection and real-time access, Prezant said. For example, a computerized, online questionnaire was developed predisaster as part of the regular annual monitoring exams for firefighters, and within 4 weeks after 9/11, FDNY was able to change the entire monitoring exam to focus on WTC. Questions were designed so that the introductory phrase could be changed with a single-stroke command. In 2000, the phrase was "during your career of firefighting have you ever…." or "in the last 12 months have you ever…." Between 9/11/01 and 10/01/01, the phrases were changed to "after the World Trade Center…." When FDNY was deployed to assist with the Hurricane Katrina response, the phrase was changed to "after Hurricane Katrina…."

The use of validated questionnaires is essential, but they are not as validated as we think, suggested Prezant. Many of them have not been studied in different populations, and almost none have been studied in a disaster population. Questionnaires may have been validated for one disease, but disasters cause multiple diseases. Using multiple, different validated disease-set questionnaires can lead to additional concerns. Concerns may be attention deficit after answering too many questions, confusion with different time spans for answers to questions (e.g., "in the last 4 weeks have you…." or "in the last 3 months...."), or similar questions in each disease set that reduce specificity of the answers.

Prezant described the World Trade Center Health Program and how it monitors and assesses firefighters. The same day that data are collected and assessed, firefighters are informed of recommended treatment or referral options. Prezant noted that FDNY cannot force firefighters to do the follow-up, but they make it free (through their health benefits program) and as easy as possible to get mental health treatment, physical health treatment, medications, benefits counseling, and so on.

IRB Processes

FDNY leverages preexisting IRB relationships for rapid review in a disaster. In addition, as long as the questionnaires, tests, and interventions (if any) are standards of care that the local health care entity was going to do anyway, then the IRB is often willing to review only the analytic portion. Prezant expressed support for a national IRB. A concern highlighted by Prezant is that many IRBs still do not understand, or have little experience with, the Federal Confidentiality Certificate. Also, consent forms typically state that the researchers and their institutions are not responsible for any complications the subject may directly or indirectly suffer from the testing protocol. Unless this line is removed, he said, most workers will not sign this consent because they correctly or incorrectly presume they are giving up their rights to workers' compensation and any litigation for damages.

Focusing on the Human Need to Help

Prezant stressed that the goal of research in response to a disaster is not just to record events, determine mechanisms and outcomes, and design interventions, although all of these are essential to response. The most important goal after a disaster, and the one required for all of the above to be possible, is to stimulate human decency, he said, by focusing on our natural impulse to reach out and help people and building a lasting relationship where at first there was only the desire and the urgency to help, and not the established scientific need to help.

HURRICANE KATRINA

Although Hurricane Katrina occurred nearly a decade ago in August 2005, it was such an enormous storm, affecting such a large geographic area and impacting so many lives, that remnants of the phenomenal amount of damage are still apparent today. Katrina had a huge effect on many different systems, including critical infrastructure, health, education, and community systems, said David Abramson, deputy director of the National Center for Disaster Preparedness at Columbia University. Abramson shared his perspectives on engaging in rapid research based on his experiences during and after Hurricane Katrina.

Gulf Coast Child and Family Health Study

Abramson elaborated on one of the larger community-based studies in which he participated, the Gulf Coast Child and Family Health Study, begun in 2006 and funded through the Children's Health Fund and the Merck Foundation. The study focused on identifying health and social service needs among this displaced and heavily impacted population. Data were collected from 1,079 randomly sampled households over the span of 29 days for the start of a 5-year longitudinal study. The sample was intended to represent 60,000 to 100,000 displaced and/or heavily affected Katrina survivors.

The immediate challenges in operationalizing this study were enormous, Abramson said. Even though he and his colleagues started working on a protocol just a few weeks after the storm, the first barrier was access to sample frame data (or the set of information used to identify the population for research). Namely they were looking for information on where the displaced populations were, especially congregate settings to help frame their research protocol. FEMA was managing the congregate settings population and had meticulous data, he said, but they did not release any of it for his research. A second challenge, Abramson added, was that the sampling frame was a moving target after they got the initial access. For example, by the time the protocol was approved, FEMA had triggered its deadline for evacuees to leave the hotels, so identifying and locating participants had to be done all over again. Another challenge they anticipated was whether or not researchers would be able to gain access to these public and private sites once they found them. Time was the biggest issue, as it becomes more difficult to find people as time passes and recall bias can increase over time. Abramson said there was no reliable Internet access in many places they went, and to account for that anticipated challenge they developed field management databases for tablets that can batch data and upload later when an Internet connection is available. Researchers were also sure to have pens and hard copies of the survey they were administering.

To quicken the time line and mobilize the research infrastructure more rapidly, Abramson used the infrastructure and expertise he already had in place for an HIV longitudinal cohort study happening in the New York City metropolitan area. This existing infrastructure offered Abramson and his team rapid access to data systems, qualified interviewers, research staff, staff knowledge of working with vulnerable and elusive populations, and a common methodology for building and maintaining a longitudinal cohort using multistage, stratified sampling strategies. Building these elements from scratch would have delayed the time line and kept them from getting into the field as quickly as possible to capture the ephemeral data. In addition, Abramson was connected with more than 25 graduate students who were interested in coming to the Gulf Coast to conduct the research. Although this worked as a great model in this case, it may be difficult to fund this type of "attaching" to an existing research infrastructure as a sustainable future model for disaster research. Standardizing that process across institutions nationwide that are interested in disaster research may be a challenge as well, but in cases where relationships are already built, it may also be very efficient.

By the time they were ready for the IRB submission, it was approximately 4 months after the storm hit. The IRB understood the need for speed in this case and provided a rapid expedited review. The process involved a back-and-forth dialogue and helped to establish a relationship that is now in place to facilitate rapid IRB approval in future disasters. Upon initial submission, the head of Columbia University Medical Center's IRB informed Abramson that his protocol for the Gulf Coast Child and Family Health Study would need to consider additional elements: addressing the vulnerability of the subjects; systematic referral of subjects to care; ability to identify crises as they occur; endorsement from the community or government; the safety, training, and preparation of the field team; and compliance with local "Duty to Report" laws regarding abuse and neglect (which may differ by state). Agreeing that these items were important and needed to be examined, they were added to the protocol. The IRB director and chairs ultimately granted approval days before Abramson was to enter the field, and they now have an understanding of the time line importance for certain disaster-related projects. If an IRB is not as understanding and flexible as the one in this case, this could be another potentially vulnerable area for a researcher's time line, especially in the case of multiple institutions working together and needing approval by separate IRBs. Education and sharing of disaster-related research projects at IRB forums and net-working events could be a way to shift perception of the IRBs from a barrier to a partner.

Engaging and Leveraging Existing Partners

Throughout the discussions, various participants noted the importance of building and sustaining relationships with organizations on the ground and local to the affected community. The Gulf Coast Child and Family Health Study was fortunate to leverage partners of their home institution for resources, but also those local partners who were familiar with the community. Local partnerships can aid in efficiency as well as facilitate the "returning of data" back to the community to help them in making informed changes and future decisions. Abramson noted that a critical partner in achieving their rapid mobilization was the Children's Health Fund, which already had clinical teams deployed in the field, having sent some of their mobile medical units to the Gulf for what they dubbed "Operation Assist," and had existing connections with state and local officials. The Children's Health Fund also had a stable funding mechanism, having raised $10 million to $15 million under the banner of Operation Assist, and was willing to share one of their mobile units as a public health field office. Trying to raise funds to support a mobile office and spend the time to make connections with government officials would have again delayed the research back even further. Abramson explained that the 35-foot-long mobile unit, branded with the Columbia University and Children's Health Fund names and logos and set up inside with the necessary office equipment, was a centerpiece of the operation because of the branding of the mobile unit and the researchers (through the ID badges and distinctive tote bags and hats). This was a key element of success as the community became familiar with the project, and it offered an element of legitimacy.

Highlighting the need to connect with local institutions, Abramson said that the Louisiana Department of Health and Hospital was also a critical partner, endorsing the study, offering resources and assistance, and importantly, providing official Louisiana Department of Health and Hospital badges for researchers that helped to enable access to the trailer parks and other congregate settings. Abramson noted that for the Gulf study, this relationship with the Louisiana Department of Health and Hospital was more casual, and he would share research findings on occasion. Looking back, he realized it should have been more formalized, so for the more recent Hurricane Sandy Child and Family Health Study, he created the Public Partnership Group to make a more formal connection with the state agencies in New Jersey. This group is composed of the health department, children and families, and human services within the state, and has a more formal reporting structure so it will receive the data from the field within weeks to make sure it is actionable for policy and programmatic purposes. With mobile and electronic tools and resources they did not have during the Gulf Coast

Child and Family Health Study, they are actually now able to send data to their partners daily when available, making it possible for policy decisions to be made more quickly with more information. Having research teams connected as part of the formal response and recovery infrastructure could be a key method for connecting researchers and public health practice, sustain newly made relationships among partners, and elevate the significance of disaster research.

The results of the study first appeared on the front page of *The New York Times* and succeeded in calling attention to some of the unresolved issues in the Gulf following the storm that had not been appearing in national news. This galvanized the researchers, he said, because "we realized the impact we can have if we can get our research out and disseminate it widely." While Abramson first encountered several difficulties in mobilizing a research team and identifying and sustaining a cohort for their work, this singular example illustrates the reach that disaster research could potentially have on future policy decisions, recovery funding, and informed research in the next disaster.

DEEPWATER HORIZON OIL SPILL

Shortly after the Deepwater Horizon oil spill in April 2010, NIH Director Francis Collins pledged $10 million in NIH funding to initiate the Gulf Long-term Follow-up (GuLF) Study, in which NIEHS is conducting research on the health impacts of the spill on workers and volunteers cleaning it up, said Birnbaum of NIEHS. Related NIEHS programs include Deepwater Horizon Research Consortia (an extramural consortium focusing on women and children, pregnancy issues, seafood safety, and resiliency of communities); toxicology research on the compounds involved (crude oil, dispersants, polyaromatic breakdown products); and worker training for people involved in the cleanup, provided through the NIEHS Worker Education and Training Program. Birnbaum noted that although many professionals were well trained in cleanup of oil spills, many volunteers were not (e.g., college students, housewives, un-employed). Within 2 weeks of the spill, NIEHS was distributing pocket-sized safety and health awareness booklets to the cleanup workers in English, Spanish, and Vietnamese.

A Transient Study Population

Key among the challenges to conducting oil spill research was working with the atypical study population of workers and volunteers. To identify potential study participants, NIOSH was able to provide a roster of 50,000 people who were involved, and the National Guard and the Coast Guard were able to provide lists of people involved in cleanup in some way. After many negotiations, British Petroleum (BP) also provided a list of more than 130,000 workers. NIH had hoped to recruit 50,000 people to assist in cleanup, but Birnbaum said it has been extremely challenging to recruit the 33,000 enrolled thus far. About 20 percent of the workers came from out of state and then dispersed, making it difficult to find them.

Timing Sensitivity

Although the intramural study development process was fairly rapid (the new study was developed, received the necessary approvals, and researchers were in field within 10 months after the event and 8 months from the time of funding), we need to be able to do research in a disaster situation from the start, Birnbaum said. Echoing Lurie's concerns, she said waiting 8 months to 1 year later means missing baseline and peak exposure data collection and studying mid-term rather than acute effects. Awarding NIH extramural grants takes even longer: usually 12 to 14 months elapse from the time of request for funding opportunities until the actual grants are received and funded. NIH was able to fund the extramural consortium within 8 months, but in most cases individual IRB and other necessary approvals added significant time, making it 18 to 20 months from the time of the spill for most of the extramural grantees to begin to recruit for their studies. Following a more nimble NSF model Abramson mentioned, where smaller amounts of money can be disbursed more quickly, could help to address this, as well as streamlining the IRB process so researchers do not have to gather approvals with different requirements.

True baseline preexposure data were available for only a small fraction of the cohort (e.g., those from the Coast Guard), and Birnbaum suggested the need for baseline data and biospecimen collection from people who are rostered to work in a disaster cleanup. In addition, while there was a great deal of exposure data collected by BP and multiple federal and state agencies, the databases are not integrated, and Birnbaum said it has taken significant time and resources to reconstruct exposures at different places and times during the cleanup.

Summarizing the lessons learned from the NIEHS experience with the Deepwater Horizon oil spill, Birnbaum said that in a disaster, in addition to the normal occupational cohort for the site, there may be National Guard and other servicemen and women, firefighters and police officers, volunteers, and other workers involved in the response, as well as local residents whose lives and livelihoods are impacted (e.g., Gulf fishermen). Birnbaum stressed the importance of rapid and ongoing communication with all of the stakeholders, including community groups, academic partners, and industrial partners. She also noted the need to develop better capabilities to rapidly evaluate the toxicity of the exposures.

Howard of NIOSH at CDC added that NIOSH has done extensive intramural research on the Deepwater Horizon disaster from the perspective of worker safety, and referred participants to recent articles for further details (Decker et al., 2013a,b; King and Gibbons, 2011; Kitt et al., 2012; Michaels and Howard, 2012; NIOSH, 2011).

HURRICANE SANDY

Lewis Goldfrank, professor in the Department of Emergency Medicine at New York University (NYU) School of Medicine, described his research experience in New York City following Hurricane Sandy. Decisions made in each event must balance all of the stakeholders' concerns (e.g., ethical, legal, practical, organizational, social, clinical), he stated. It is also important to understand whether the actions of the communities are based on societal need or scientific, political, or economic considerations. He added that providers and investigators in a hospital or university are also part of the impacted community, and in participatory action research, the study team members may find that they are both participants and investigators. This can be an asset, as the investigators already know the community they are studying, have existing relationships with other organizations, and can see past surface data, but it could also be a potential challenge if the investigators have been directly impacted by the disaster and may be more emotionally biased.

In the face of a disaster, decisions must be made regarding how best to spend fixed research resources (money, time, effort), both to salvage existing research affected by the disaster (including cell lines, animals, specialty chemicals, antibodies, equipment, laboratories) and to initiate new research regarding the disaster. That said, if there is no IRB, no human capital, and no electronic infrastructure following the disaster, then even those stakeholders familiar with the research proposal process will find it difficult to initiate or operationalize a new proposal in the traditional sense, Goldfrank noted.

Goldfrank shared several examples of NYU research following Hurricane Sandy to illustrate his points about community. One study of outcomes among buprenorphine-naloxone[1] primary care patients after Sandy found only minimal increases in self-reported substance abuse. Goldfrank attributed this, in part, to the fact that the providers/investigators were closely linked with the community and deeply involved in the continuity of care of their patients (Tofighi et al., 2014). He also cited two rapid response studies looking at gasoline and carbon monoxide exposures; he said the studies were possible only because the NYU School of Medicine faculty and fellows are embedded in the public health infrastructure with joint institutional appointments and commitments (Chen et al., 2013; Kim et al., 2013).

Dissemination

NYU researchers are also considering mechanisms for rapid dissemination of experiential learning in a disaster (Laskowski et al., 2013). Goldfrank noted that the traditional peer-review process impeded speedy publication of Sandy research results. He raised several questions for discussion: Should there be "disaster standards" for publication with regard to rigor, methodology, response rate, control groups, etc.? Does the public good of disaster research demand open access, and if so, who funds this? Who is the author, the investigator, or the participants? Do disciplines not traditionally associated with health care delivery achieve larger importance in the face of disaster (e.g., materials science, water and sanitary engineering) and can they be cosupported?

---

[1]Buprenorphine (Subutex) and buprenorphine and naloxone (Suboxone) are used to treat opioid dependence (addiction to opioid drugs, including heroin and narcotic painkillers). Buprenorphine alone and the combination of buprenorphine and naloxone prevent withdrawal symptoms when someone stops taking opioid drugs by producing similar effects to these drugs.

The Impact of Disasters on Hospitals and Health Care

There were many questions about the role of hospitals, emergency departments, and ambulatory care units in meeting the needs of the community during the crisis, and Goldfrank said most decisions on these questions were made in "an evidence-free zone" where guidance from other disasters would have been helpful. While these issues were debated, health care clinical deficits continued or were exacerbated. Goldfrank raised concerns about the ability of a city or state to respond to a disaster without total integration of the health care system. He explained that in evacuating the hospitals, all private staff were sent to other private hospitals, public hospital personnel were sent to other public hospitals, and U.S. Department of Veterans Affairs (VA) staff were sent to other VA facilities. Because there was no universal credentialing, and it can take 2 or 3 days for a provider to be credentialed in another hospital, many would go and wait, unable to deliver care. Goldfrank suggested that staffing with providers from closed hospitals benefits the other hospitals because then they do not have to pay overtime to their staff to have the necessary coverage.

With the above issues in mind, NYU is working on a project funded by an ASPR Recovery Grant to study the impact of a major adverse climate event on health system care and development of disaster response- and resilience-based metrics. The study will examine the comparative effectiveness of adaptive options (e.g., setting up an ambulatory care center or freestanding emergency department) and the decision making necessary for the entire health community to function.

Response Research Networks

Goldfrank supported the calls for the establishment of a broader medical and public health emergency response research network locally and nationally. This network would, for example, initiate continuous meaningful relationships at all levels; facilitate data sharing for immediate and long-term collaboration; define critical research needs, priorities, and obstacles; and consider the roles of embedded researchers in disaster response. A national network could provide priority funding to support laboratory, clinical, public health, and social science studies of public health emergencies that are not adequately addressed; establish the necessary infrastructure to support research; and develop rigorous evidence-based research protocols and implementation plans for studies in anticipation of disaster.

Disasters consume health services in nontraditional ways. Where people can get care changes when the bridges or tunnels are closed, or when, for example, dialysis centers do not have power or generators. Interhospital collaborations are essential to support resiliency in a community and facilitate better research networks, Goldfrank continued. There have been numerous joint preparedness ventures among New York City public, private, and VA hospitals, and university and hospital affiliations move faculty and residents back and forth among hospitals, strengthening intellectual collaboration. The Poison Control Center and the Office of the Chief Medical Examiner are also key collaborators in research.

SHARED LESSONS ACROSS DISASTERS

Across the case presentations, some speakers highlighted the need to get into the field rapidly and immediately start collecting what Abramson referred to as "ephemeral data." These baseline data can quickly disappear (e.g., toxin levels dissipate, people cannot be located for specimen collection, personal recall bias increases over time for a variety of intentional and unintentional reasons). In addition, structural and cultural barriers encountered during research attempts following disasters make it difficult to accomplish the goal of a robust science response. However, recent progress made in emergency planning and community resilience building lends possibilities for research to succeed.

Removing Structural Barriers

A few participants discussed further the need to address critical structural barriers and build better systems for everyday use that can be scaled up in a disaster, rather than focusing on building systems just for use in disasters. Goldfrank stressed the importance of being able to deliver everyday health care to everyone and opined that we "will not achieve excellence, as we would consider acceptable, unless we accomplish universal health care." Prezant added that before the disaster, there need to be opportunities to develop relationships that can be translated into an improved health care infrastructure when needed (discussed further on page 39).

Abramson raised the issue of silos and proprietary data systems as barriers to disaster research. Many entities (e.g., FEMA, U.S. Department of Homeland Security, other emergency management) create their own data systems to facilitate their work and become very protective of their data, systems, and projects, making interoperability before and during an incident a challenge. Some even seem unwilling to acknowledge that data they are collecting could be very helpful to the community at large. Abramson noted that this goes beyond academic researchers seeking access, and he has heard from local and state health officials who could not access government datasets to help facilitate their work. At the local level the silos of information can also trickle down, making it difficult for local health departments, hospitals, and emergency ma-nagement agencies to easily talk and share data across sectors. A part-icipant noted the potential for a symbiotic relationship between local health departments and researchers. The resources and people that local health departments can pool can be beneficial to researchers, and the information that researchers generate can be beneficial to local health departments.

Prezant highlighted the need for funding streams for preparedness research and called for data-driven advocacy to establish and maintain credibility of the field after the initial emotional funding response subsides. Disaster response research cannot compete in the process as it exists now; for example, there is not time to write extensive proposals, the proper control groups are not always possible, and there are numerous simultaneous, and often unknown, confounders. We need to change the expectations of federal funding agencies with regard to disaster response research, he said.

Building Coalitions and Goodwill in Advance

A discussion point throughout the case studies was the benefit that could be realized in getting different groups to work together to prepare and develop "prepositioned goodwill" that can help them to be ready to work together in a disaster. Abramson highlighted the role of health care coalitions in getting hospitals to begin to work together and noted the need to broaden those coalitions so they begin to engage other health care providers within a larger health system and then the community stakeholder groups. Prezant commented that each area has its own challenges for developing networks. In a real disaster, many barriers tend to disappear for the first few days, but then they recur. In some cases excellence can be a barrier, as expert entities do not want to make compromises. In other cases there may be little or no structure to begin with, making it difficult to develop any sort of network. What is needed is a solid public health infrastructure, because without a foundation for everyday medicine, there is no foundation for disaster medicine, he said.

Engaging the Community

The concept of developing prepositioned goodwill was discussed further with specific focus on engaging the community as both participants and partners in disaster research. It was noted that there are often misunderstandings about how research is used, in part because of the lack of dissemination of the findings to community members whose data were used. This can lead to a lack of trust of research and researchers. Abramson advocated for going back into the community with data in hand to talk about the findings in a direct and real way, so that the community can begin to have ownership over the findings. The community can also add perspective to the findings and will have a far better idea of potential causal mechanisms and relationships, he said. (This concept is further elaborated on in Chapter 5.) He acknowledged that it is very labor intensive, but if researchers plan to go into a community to begin research, they have to be committed to going back in after the study is done to share the data in a reasonable time frame.

Managing, defining, and redefining expectations is important, Prezant said, both our own expectations as well as the community's. Repairing damage done in the past that has created this distrust may not be possible, but it is possible and essential to avoid causing further damage in the future. Abramson added that emergency preparedness gives public health the opportunity to partner with emergency management and community-based groups to bring marginalized populations to the table to talk about how disasters affect all of us and begin to empower different elements within the community. Later, when public health wants to engage them in other chronic issues—smoking, alcohol, nutrition, obesity—relationships are already built. This can operate in the reverse as well, as communities may identify needs they prioritize that affect them every day, and engaging them in those areas first could prove beneficial to later discussions about disaster research.

The next several chapters highlight the issues and ongoing progress by stakeholders within each of the identified key areas. Some discussions revolved around regulatory and standardization issues, such as facilitating a central IRB or creating funding mechanisms to be deployed. Others brought in important cultural conversations about communities—engaging the communities in this type of research and promoting citizen science. Concluding each section is a compilation of top items relative to the challenges and issues, opportunities for improvement, and critical partnerships and collaborations necessary to advance research response capabilities.

4

Addressing Institutional Review Board Barriers to Health Research Implementation

The barriers that IRBs present to researchers following a disaster are broad and complex and often can delay a study getting off the ground. Participants explored strategies to balance human subject protections while enabling timely IRB review of research protocols, discussed options to obtain informed consent in emergency situations, and considered the ethics of data collection for special populations in disasters.

THE PUBLIC HEALTH EMERGENCY RESEARCH REVIEW BOARD

In 2011, the National Preparedness and Research Science Board (NPRSB)[1] at ASPR produced a report on science preparedness disaster research, discussing what would be needed to bring the ongoing efforts by NIH, CDC, ASPR, and others together in a more cohesive and organized way.[2] Among its recommendations, the NPRSB called for the creation of a PHERRB, an IRB that would be able to rapidly convene to assess research protocols while maintaining very robust protections for human subjects. Diane DiEuliis, deputy director of the Office of Policy and Planning at ASPR, said that ASPR has been working with NIH to develop the PHERRB. It was established in 2012 by HHS and is main-

[1]Formerly the National Biodefense Science Board.

[2]Available at http://www.phe.gov/Preparedness/legal/boards/nprsb/Documents/nbsbrec14.pdf (accessed September 8, 2014).

tained by NIH through the Office of Human Subjects Research Protections (OHSRP).

Michael Gottesman, deputy director for intramural research at NIH and the institutional official at NIH responsible for OHSRP, said NIH has experience in conducting research under disaster conditions (e.g., the GuLF Study discussed by Birnbaum). In addition, NIH has an extensive IRB system, many reliance agreements and cooperative relations with the IRBs throughout the country, and numerous experts at its disposal. As host of the PHERRB, NIH provides staff, develops operating procedures, and maintains operations.

The PHERRB is a central IRB and serves as the single IRB for human subjects protections review of HHS-conducted, -supported, or -regulated research studies addressing public health emergencies (e.g., natural disasters, biohazards including anthrax, chemical and radiological emergencies, oil spills, pandemic influenza or other infectious diseases, and other mass casualty events). Gottesman explained that the PHERRB would provide human subjects protections/regulatory review only under existing applicable federal regulations (including 45 CFR 46 and/or 21 CFR 50 and 56). The PHERRB can serve as the IRB of record for any institution (this can be a state health department, an academic medical center, a community hospital, etc.) that is engaged in the conduct of the protocol and that executes a reliance agreement with NIH for PHERRB review. At present, use of the PHERRB is generally encouraged but not required, so institutions conducting public health emergency research could choose to use a local IRB (or multiple IRBs) for human subject protections review. The PHERRB would conduct initial reviews, continuing reviews, review of amendments, review of unanticipated problems, and local context review. Gottesman noted that review by the PHERRB does not replace other institutional oversight responsibilities (e.g., principal investigator training, adequacy of local resources, ancillary reviews, IRB office functions).

An IRB Authorization Agreement (reliance agreement) between NIH and the institution conducting the research is required. The reliance agreement allows the PHERRB to conduct human subjects research protections review of a public health emergency research protocol in the place of an IRB in a local community, under the NIH Federal-wide Assurance.[3] The agreement provides a road map for the life of the study and the reliance relationship. It also helps institutions consider all issues

---

[3]See http://www.hhs.gov/ohrp/assurances/assurances/filasurt.html (accessed November 10, 2014).

in advance and describes the division of responsibilities between the PHERRB and the local institution (e.g., conflict of interest, investigator human subjects protection training, confidentiality and privacy, compensation of participants, other committee reviews that may be needed). Gottesman noted that NIH currently has 12 IRBs, and any of them can be designated to serve as the PHERRB IRB of record. In addition, NIH is prepared to assemble an IRB as needed to deal with multicomponent disasters (i.e., additional expertise could be brought into any of the basic IRBs). In general, principal investigators would be able to access the presubmission application, frequently asked questions, and other information about the PHERRB process on the OHSRP website. Upon submission of a protocol, NIH will determine if it is within the scope of PHERRB review.

One issue yet to be resolved is whether and with whom reliance agreements should be prenegotiated. Another question is whether individual academic institutions would want to have these open-ended reliance agreements. Could protocols be developed in advance of an emergency to accelerate initiation of research activities, and if so, would these protocols be developed by NIH, or would NIH solicit submissions? Gottesman noted that the concern with soliciting submissions is that there could be hundreds or even thousands of protocols, and the IRB system would come to a crashing halt. NIH could perhaps solicit protocols from a limited number of institutions, those that are part of a clinical research network or are highly likely in some other way to have to deal with emergencies.

STATE HEALTH DEPARTMENT IRB PERSPECTIVE

Nell Allbritton, the IRB director for the Louisiana Department of Health and Hospitals, said her experience shows that a state agency has a set of concerns that are very different from those of researchers and universities. A key issue for a state health department is patient privacy. The state errs on the side of caution when allowing researchers access to patients, she said. In addition, transitional staff and space during disaster response can compromise the security of confidential data and the privacy of subjects. The first priority for a public health agency is to respond and to mobilize quickly so that patients are removed from harm and continue to receive services. Monitoring or assisting in research efforts can be a strain on the resources of the health department and its ability to be responsive to the community's needs. Another concern for the health department is that research participants will confuse research for clinical services (referred to as therapeutic misconception). Communities decimated by disaster are also vulnerable to exploitation and additional harm. Research can be designed to pose minimal risk to participants, but could still compromise the community's ability to respond and recover. Finally, maintaining the participation of the population being studied is a challenge for disaster research, as survivors relocate and might lose access to prior means of communication.

Recent Proposals in Louisiana

Allbritton shared several examples of disaster research proposals that her IRB has dealt with in recent years. The first example from 2005–2006 involved a Louisiana State University study to evaluate rapid-needs assessments conducted by the state mental health services provider. Around 250,000 people were displaced to Baton Rouge following Hurricane Katrina, and more than 6,000 people who sought treatment at the Capital Area Human Services District were surveyed with informed consent. However, the study had not been reviewed or approved by the IRB, Allbritton said. The health department learned of the study prior to publication and would not let its publication proceed until the IRB had reviewed the manuscript. (She clarified that while it is possible that the study was approved by the university IRB, the state IRB is the IRB of record because a state mental health services population was the study population.) Another Louisiana State University research project, examining the efficacy of a group treatment protocol for posttraumatic stress disorder, was able to modify its existing protocol for use with Hurricane Katrina survivors. The IRB turnaround was rapid, as this was a modification of research already being done.

In 2009, Tulane University sought to identify the most effective therapy model for stress reduction of substance-abusing adults in disaster-prone regions. The intent was to study clients who entered addictive disorders clinics, correlated to periods of natural disaster that occurred in the region. The instruments and the methodology were submitted and approved by the IRB prior to the commencement of the study period, Allbritton said. As it turned out, there was no hurricane activity in 2009 in the region, so while this is a model of preapproval of a protocol, the research did not occur. More recently, the IRB approved a

Tulane University study comparing mental and physical health outcomes over a 4-year period in 1,800 women exposed in varying degrees to the Deepwater Horizon disaster.

Lessons in Reviewing Disaster Proposals

Drawing on her experience with these four studies as well as others, Allbritton shared some of the lessons learned by the IRB. The oil spill study, in particular, raised the issue of therapeutic misconception, she said. The IRB ensured that the consent forms clearly defined what would be done with the blood and saliva samples so that none of the participants would mistake consenting to give samples for being able to receive clinical services. Investigators are responsible for assessing individual decisional capacity and the possible effects of the research on participants, and Allbritton added that monetary incentives can be coercive. In a disaster situation, investigators or support staff should be trained to identify participants who are distressed and need aid, and refer them for care. There should also be a plan for care of researchers exposed to emotionally difficult situations. Including community leadership in the IRB review of a protocol is the best way to get community buy-in before the protocol is deployed, Allbritton said. Preapproval of the protocol and methodology expedites deployment of the study, and provisions for confidentiality and privacy should be an explicit part of the research plan. Ground-level program staff must also be prepared to redirect researchers to the IRB for approval of any deviations from the protocol.

With regard to reliance agreements, Allbritton noted that there is currently language in the Louisiana state rule that prohibits reliance agreements with other IRBs and would therefore prevent reliance agreements with the PHERRB. However, she agreed to return to her state and bring up the need to consider working with the PHERRB or a centralized IRB.

While there is not a separate or unique application process for disaster protocol IRB review, there are extra questions that the IRB for the Louisiana Department of Health and Hospitals recommends researchers consider in developing their protocol and methodology (see Box 4-1). Often, the IRB might approve a protocol with stipulations that certain changes be made, and this delays the process as researchers must then return to the IRB with the answers to the questions. Where applicable, including answers to these questions in the protocol will hopefully reduce the revisions that the IRB requires, Allbritton said.

Disaster takes us out of routine, Allbritton concluded. As a state agency, day-to-day operations change completely, and employees may also be directly impacted. Maintaining services is challenging, as even normal activities require additional oversight. The research component of the department, unfortunately, does not take priority in times of crisis, but it is important not to discourage or prevent this kind of work from being done. Therefore, Allbritton said, the state IRB must employ additional measures to ensure proper protections for public health consumers participating in postdisaster research and safeguard the ability of the department to maintain the standard operating level during catastrophic events.

BOX 4-1
Questions to Address for Institutional Review Board Review of a Disaster Protocol from Nell Allbritton

- Does the design make it easy to collect data immediately after the disaster occurs?
- Do the researchers contribute their time in relief efforts in addition to collecting data?
- Are the researchers prepared to convince disaster relief workers that the study is beneficial to the survivors in order to gain access to participants?
- Does the protocol account for continuing research and recruitment during and after the relocation of survivors?
- Will researchers ask participants for contact information to be shared from agencies as part of informed consent?
- What alternative resources will the researchers provide to participants?
- Do consent forms account for diversity in age, culture, and education?
- How will the researchers determine who may give consent for minors to participate?
- Has the community given consent?

SOURCE: Allbritton presentation, June 13, 2014.

ETHICS, OVERSIGHT, AND CONDUCT OF POSTDISASTER RESEARCH

Given the priority of meeting the immediate medical and mental health needs of survivors of and witnesses to a disaster, the issue of deciding when and how to conduct mental and behavioral health research with these populations is logistically and ethically challenging, said Holly Taylor, core faculty at the Johns Hopkins Berman Institute of Bioethics. With funding from the Preparedness and Emergency Response Center (a CDC-funded entity) at the Johns Hopkins Bloomberg School of Public Health, Taylor set out to describe and consider the ethical challenges encountered by IRBs and investigators in the review, oversight, and conduct of postdisaster research.

The study is ongoing, but Taylor was able to share some of her preliminary findings. She noted that the IRBs managed reviews of disaster research in many ways. In some cases, a unique committee or the IRB subcommittee was created to review the study prior to the IRB review, and it appeared to look at issues unrelated to human subjects research. Some IRBs put the disaster protocols into the routine review process, while others prioritized them.

Among the concerns raised by the IRB members she interviewed were the quality of the research proposed and the feeling that researchers were "following the money." The level of harm to which subjects may be exposed was also a concern (however, Taylor added that the current literature strongly indicates that people do not experience any additional harm as a result of being interviewed). The IRB members also raised concerns about the burden on subjects, potential for therapeutic misconception, and safety of research staff. Challenges encountered by the IRBs interviewed included the speed required, the multiple stakeholders involved (including labor unions and employers when workplaces are involved, as well as law enforcement and the legal system if it is a crime scene), lack of coordination among institutions and the IRBs, turf battles with affiliated institutions, multisite research, and the value of certificates of confidentiality (especially relative to federal court cases).

The principal investigators interviewed reported positive experience with the IRBs (with the exception of navigating multiple IRBs). Investigators reported that the IRBs had issues with the quality of the research they proposed, asked them about the level of harm to which subjects need to be exposed, and stressed the importance of having appropriate referrals in place. Procedural challenges highlighted by investigators included funding, additional layers of review, lack of communication among federal sponsors, and access to populations. Substantive challenges mentioned by investigators were the availability of appropriate services for referral (which are often lacking in a disaster) and the potential vulnerability of the subjects.

Some unique challenges were noted. For example, there is community-wide impact, and the affected population may include the study teams. There are also infrastructure issues impacting the retention and follow-up of displaced subjects. Local staff at local agencies are overwhelmed, and it is challenging to train them to adopt new interventions while they are managing their own personal and professional priorities. The number of medical service providers, social service providers, agency staff, and other research teams in the field created confusion for the subjects. Taylor explained that this became a problem for one research team when they were mistaken for a different research team that had apparently made promises they did not fulfill. DiEuliis added that after Hurricane Sandy, one issue raised by investigators was the potential for "survey fatigue" among participants, given the large number of research projects being done concurrently. It was suggested that CDC, NIH, FEMA, ASPR, and other relevant agencies could coordinate somehow so that all of the investigators could see each other's survey populations and questions. She noted that ASPR, working with NIEHS, has been building a web space for the grantees that will have a map and listing of shared research populations. The next step is working with the investigators to determine the best way to help them coordinate with each other. She suggested that the PHERRB may be able to provide assistance in this area.

CHALLENGES AND OPPORTUNITIES

DiEuliis reported on the top challenges and issues identified by participants (see Box 4-2). She indicated that there was broad recognition of the usefulness of having a national-level, centralized IRB, such as the PHERRB. Research during a disaster is different from general research, and the use of a central IRB in a disaster is not commonplace.

Another issue raised was the need for coordination among in-stitutions, the IRBs, and the federal entities funding the research. It

BOX 4-2
Addressing IRB Barriers to Health Research Implementation[a]
Challenges and Issues

- Recognition of the usefulness of the PHERRB, but also that there would be same standards for disaster research.
- Coordination among institutions/the IRBs/federal support entities, particularly with regard to "survey fatigue" in affected populations.
- Quality of research and asking the most important questions.
- Differentiation of acute needs (at beginning of an outbreak) versus longer term, more structured clinical studies; are definitions needed?
- Reliance agreements and how to approach them. Acknowledgment that states may not recognize these.
- Confusion of "research" versus "services."

Critical Partnerships and Collaborations

- States, localities, research institutions, principal investigators, federal agencies.

[a]The challenges, opportunities, and partnerships listed were identified by one or more individual participants in this breakout panel discussion. This summary was prepared by the panel facilitator and presented in the subsequent plenary session. This list is not meant to reflect a consensus among workshop participants.

SOURCE: Plenary session summary of breakout panel discussion as reported by panel facilitator Diane DiEuliis.

was suggested that the absence of coordination could lead to survey fatigue in affected populations, with many different investigators approaching the same people or populations for different study protocols. During the discussion, a participant suggested that the central IRB could maintain a list of all disaster-related protocols and make the list available to all researchers and the IRB reviewers. Several participants highlighted the importance of understanding what is acceptable to the community in terms of human subjects protection (an example given was a tribal entity that had very different views of who should have access to their data and how that data could be profiled and published). This may mean involving the community in developing the protocol for the IRB submission.

With regard to approval and coordination of the many potential research studies, a participant stated that it can be difficult to make the distinction between an investigator who is clearly taking advantage of a situation (i.e., "following the funding") versus one who sees a real connection to his or her ongoing work. DiEuliis pointed out that a stipulation of the Hurricane Sandy supplemental funding was that any outside institutions (outside of the hurricane-affected states) seeking funding needed to demonstrate that they had relationships in the communities and with the affected populations. Taylor suggested looking at how the IRBs handle international collaborations for lessons that could be applied to working with investigators from outside the disaster-affected area (e.g., requiring documentation that researchers are collaborating with a particular local organization and have the IRB review from the local level). A participant referred others to the World Association for Disaster and Emergency Medicine updated disaster research and evaluation frameworks (Birnbaum et al., 2014), which offers five frameworks to apply to studying and comparing disasters and evaluating interventions. The critical piece of these frameworks is the inclusion of standardized definitions throughout.

In the same vein, some participants emphasized the need for attention to the quality of the research proposed. Are we asking the most important questions when looking back over the history of clinical research done during disasters, DiEuliis asked, or are we asking the same questions over again? There was also discussion of differentiation between acute needs (at the very beginning of an outbreak or event) versus long-term, more structured clinical studies. Several participants discussed the possible need for definitions or a rubric for the different kinds of research that would be needed during and after a disaster, and the associated IRB needs.

Much discussion took place about how best to approach and broker reliance agreements. It was reiterated that some states may not recognize the type of reliance agreements that would be done at the federal level directly with institutions. Several participants stressed that reliance agreements should clearly spell out the roles and responsibilities of the entities involved (e.g., HIPAA responsibility). Finally, DiEuliis said, the issue of therapeutic misconception was discussed further, including ensuring that study participants understand research versus services and why the research they might be part of is of value to recovery.

5

Partnering with the Community to Enable Research

As mentioned previously in Chapter 3, engaging the community to become involved in disaster research is a goal of many researchers, yet successful access still has many challenges. Often these are due to outside research teams unfamiliar with the communities entering after a disaster with their own agendas in mind and a lack of communication with and commitment to the people they are studying. Jack Herrmann, senior advisor and chief of public health programs at the National Association of County and City Health Officials (NACCHO), and Joseph "Chip" Hughes, program director for the Worker Education and Training Branch at NIEHS, facilitated discussion on engaging community and citizen scientists in disaster research. Participants considered strategies to strengthen the interface and collaborations with first responders and emergency management, health departments, workers, and others to promote successful disaster research.

PARTNERING FOR EPIDEMIOLOGY RESEARCH

Texas leads the nation in the number of presidentially declared disasters, said David Lakey, commissioner of the Texas Department of State Health Services (DSHS). From 2008 through 2013, response events in Texas have included, for example, Hurricanes Alex, Dolly, Eduard Gustav, and Ike; the Yearning for Zion Ranch evacuation of children from polygamist families because of abuse allegations; the West fertilizer plant explosion; wildfires; the H1N1 pandemic; West Nile virus; food-borne outbreaks; epidemiological investigations (e.g., tuberculosis, mercury poisoning from cosmetics); investigation of compounding pharmacies; and unaccompanied minors crossing the Texas–Mexico border. The Texas DSHS is responsible for the co-ordination of health and medical response.

Timely information after a disaster is essential, and Texas DSHS uses the Community Assessment for Public Health Emergency Response (CASPER) tool, an epidemiologic technique to rapidly provide low-cost, household-based information about community needs. Following a disaster, teams conduct door-to-door household surveys about public health needs and emergency management issues such as health status, access to utilities, access to health care, mental health issues, evacuation behaviors, messaging, and recovery needs. Lakey noted that the CASPER system has been critical for improvement of disaster planning and response in Texas. In response to a question about the IRB review, Lakey noted that CASPER is a tool being used in realtime to get information for disaster response improvement. This is an example of "Disaster Epidemiology," which can be done more quickly and span topic areas more widely than traditional research often does. For other questions that are longer term, full IRB approval is received beforehand. A participant added that there is a process before the survey that explains who is doing the survey, why, what they are doing, and what will be done with the results; people can then choose whether to participate.

State Health Department Research

With the goal of continuous quality improvement in mind, the Texas DSHS has published nearly 50 peer-reviewed articles on public health preparedness over the past decade, Lakey said.[1] These are written by DSHS regional and central office staff from a variety of programs, often with academic partners as coauthors. Lakey stressed the value of partnering with academia in the community, noting that Texas DSHS has collaborated with Texas A&M, University of Texas, and University of North Texas. Academic partners can help to provide baseline data, conduct studies, facilitate stakeholder meetings, provide surge capacity (e.g., staff, space for shelters), assess training needs, provide technical assistance, and collaborate on publications. Texas DSHS has also developed formal internship opportunities for students, and a residency program so that preventive medicine residents can gain experience in the

[1]See http://www.dshs.state.tx.us/commprep/publications.aspx (accessed December 12, 2014).

field of public health during a disaster. Lakey added that after-action reports are also an essential component of continuous quality improvement, but they are not always accessible to a broader audience. He shared an example of what he described as a negative research-related experience. In 2008 during Hurricane Ike, he received phone calls from people he did not know who were seeking information for articles they wanted to publish in the media. It was clear to Lakey that these requesters had obvious biases for how they planned to present their story.

Disaster Epidemiology

Lakey also shared several examples of how disaster epidemiology research has been effective and helpful in response (also discussed further in Chapter 6). A surveillance study tracking injury deaths related to Hurricane Ike was intended to identify strategies to prevent or reduce hurricane-related mortality in the future. Working with partners, data were collected from a variety of sources, including medical examiners, justices of the peace, coroners, forensic centers, hospitals, and regional epidemiologists. The majority of the 74 deaths reported were indirectly related to the hurricane, suggesting that the evacuation of people out of the disaster zone worked well. However, many succumbed to carbon monoxide poisoning in their temporary quarters (from inappropriate use of stoves and heaters) or were hit by falling trees as they tried to clear their land. This is important information for how we approach disasters, Lakey said, because it demonstrates the need to not only evacuate people, but to give them information on how they can remain healthy in the aftermath.

The epidemiological investigation of the West fertilizer plant explosion in 2013 is an example of collaborations among local, regional, state, and federal agencies. The local public health department was the lead agency, which helped to ensure that the community was involved in the research being done in their community, Lakey explained. Texas DSHS provided the technical expertise, and additional resources and best practices were shared by CDC and other agencies. Using data from the medical examiner, death certificates, hospitals, urgent care clinics, and survivor interviews, Lakey and colleagues characterized the injuries, resource needs and distribution, and communication priorities for affected individuals to help inform practice in future disasters.

Success in these cases and others is dependent on relationships. As many responders know, to be most effective, partners need to get to know each other before an event, Lakey said. This applies to disaster research as well, and he noted that, based on experience, he is very cautious about engaging with a previously unknown outside entity that appears during disaster response wanting to do research. He offered several relationship-building lessons:

- Partner early with stakeholders in the investigation-forming process to solicit expectations.
- Combine efforts to make an investigation more useful to stake-holders and maximize resources.
- Continue and expand pre-event partnerships to aid in coll-aboration during and after an incident.
- Develop nontraditional partnerships for public health (e.g., with the Texas State Fire Marshal).

In closing, Lakey said that in conducting research during disasters, it is important to partner with trusted researchers and to have clear, agreed-upon objectives, developed with input from the appropriate stakeholders (public, private, local, state, and federal). Research should be coordinated with the ICS, which can help avoid duplication of effort. There are lessons to be learned from community-based participatory research, including understanding what is important to the community and, as Abramson previously noted, the need to disseminate results back to the community. Researchers also need to be aware of the politics that may play into the overall response. Overall, be sensitive and respectful to those we are trying to serve, he concluded.

ESTABLISHING TRUST IN THE COMMUNITY

Stephen Bradberry, executive director of the Alliance Institute, expanded on the concept of maintaining an ongoing connection with the community, previously emphasized by Goldfrank during his remarks about hospital populations during Hurricane Sandy. When a disaster happens and researchers need the help of the community, Bradberry also reiterated that it is important to have trust established with the community. He pointed out that distrust comes from years of people coming into the community to collect data and then leaving, never to be heard from again. Bradberry noted that even well-intentioned researchers often focus on high-quality medical services and community-centered health homes while neglecting the community environment. The community environment has many resources, including the residents, patients, and networks, and their experience with, for example, advocacy, community meetings, and mobilizations. The community has a wealth of knowledge regarding how they, as a community, can best be engaged, and what serves their needs in their environment. The people living in a particular area are often very knowledgeable about the dangers they face by living in that region (e.g., oil leaking from wells), and about the best ways to deal with a situation, but they are rarely asked. Instead, they are given recommendations and told how things will be done, which can lead to resistance and resentment.

As an example, Bradberry recalled the comment by Birnbaum that the NIEHS GuLF Study (on the health impacts of the Deepwater Horizon oil spill) has had challenges recruiting participants and is about 20,000 participants short of its goal. Bradberry suggested this is due to "an extreme lack of trust." He said that during the community meetings when the study was outlined, the community suggested that their immediate need was for health centers because people were sick and needed care. However, that was not the path that was chosen, he said. In addition, people were aware that BP Global had full control of the media and of the recovery. They were being asked to trust NIEHS, which is part of the same government that had put the party responsible for the accident (i.e., BP) in charge of the recovery.

Regarding presentation of information to the community, Bradberry said people in the community are most interested in learning what actions they need to take. The suggested actions should be up front, he said, with the data following after for those who may be interested. This is opposite of how scientists usually present information (with data first and recommendations at the end). Including the community in the work and sharing the resulting information can alleviate many of the challenges associated with data collection and obtaining baseline information in past disasters.

PARTNERING WITH UNIONS, WORKERS' ORGANIZATIONS, AND WORKERS

Depending on the disaster setting, multiple sets of worker populations are involved, said Craig Slatin, principal investigator and director of The New England Consortium, based in the College of Health

Sciences at the University of Massachusetts Lowell. If the site is a plant (e.g., the fertilizer plant in West, Texas), facility workers may be on-site. There will also be a broad range of emergency responders; emergency management, public health, medical, and social workers; skilled support workers; workers involved in the cleanup and in construction labor; and others.

Although much of the focus in a community impacted by a disaster is on the safety and health of the residents and businesses, those involved in cleanup should be monitored as well. Recovery and remediation work is often done by low-wage workers. For example, following Hurricane Katrina, much of the work was done by immigrant day laborers. Slatin described a study conducted jointly by the University of California, Los Angeles, Labor and Occupational Safety Health program, and the National Day Laborer Organizing Network (NDLON) of health and safety issues for the Latino migrant laborers in the region. The study found that immigrant workers were gutting buildings, cleaning up debris, and tearing out moldy sheetrock from flooded houses, mostly without any protective gear. They were then going "home" after work (often an abandoned car or a shelter with nowhere to wash) to sleep in their work clothes, or paying to sleep in soaking-wet tents pitched in a muddy field at City Park, where they had to pay an extra fee to use the shower. Without this study, it is likely much of this would have gone on unnoticed. While they may not have been affected by the immediate disaster, recovery workers present an important demographic that could also benefit from environmental health monitoring to ensure they are able to safely perform their job duties.

Understanding Worker Needs and Leveraging Local Knowledge

When performing research in a community, it is important to have workers who understand the needs and nuances within that community in order to access important information, as Lakey alluded to previously, especially following a disaster. However, recruiting these types of local workers presents difficulties, so it is valuable to understand the needs workers may have throughout the process. In conducting research to evaluate the health and safety hazards affecting immigrant workers in cleanup, Tomas Aguilar from NDLON faced a variety of challenges. Those challenges included being unfamiliar with the area and dealing with initial distrust and wariness from the workers (who were facing harassment from the police, immigration agents, and other workers). Slatin relayed that Aguilar tried to supplement worker interview data by observing worksites, applying for jobs, attempting to obtain protective equipment, and generally putting himself in similar situations as the workers. He discovered that the Red Cross/FEMA site was only for local residents, so he could not get assistance. Regardless, they did not have any of the protective equipment he was seeking. A nearby relief organization also had no equipment to spare. Contractors were generally hostile and suspicious and would not talk with him, and he faced obstructions when trying to observe the worksites.

Worker Safety and Sensitivities

As another example, Slatin referred to the DR2 tabletop exercise introduced by Birnbaum in the plenary session. The activity, held at the port of Los Angeles in April 2014, was designed to develop a concept of operations for NIEHS in preparation for deployment of a disaster research team. During discussions on transition (i.e., how to sustain research efforts or undertake longer-term research), those at the exercise emphasized the need to maintain the collaboration among trainers, researchers, local and state agencies, workers, and communities. Workers and their representatives participating in the DR2 exercise cautioned that workers might be partners and help to gather information for disaster research, but they also may be at risk of retaliation for disclosing information that employers do not want disclosed. Workers are also sensitive to how the research might impact their jobs. They live in these impacted communities and want their families and community to be safe, but they also want their jobs to be secure.

During the exercise in Los Angeles, participants identified several worker/community research priorities relative to the exercise scenario (earthquake-induced tsunami leading to refinery fires): have clear knowledge of what chemicals are released and an active monitoring system to protect the health of workers and community members; ensure that workers, first responders, and community members have the appropriate protective equipment; know the health and safety issues for workers and how to appropriately train them; understand the physical and psychological impacts that the event may have on communities, response workers, and refinery workers; and create a registry of those exposed.

Slatin noted that the NIEHS Worker Education and Training Program has a network of worker trainers. These worker trainers and organized labor can assist with connecting to the community and collecting data and can help build capacity and confidence in communities.

In closing, Slatin concurred with others that a key challenge for disaster research is establishing relationships before a disaster. We do not know where disasters are going to occur, and there is not funding for the development of partnerships and relationships, Slatin added, which can be fundamental for conducting a collaborative, successful study. Based on his personal experience, it is difficult to get the support of one's institution to spend the time and resources to go into the community and build these relationships in the case that an incident occurs to precipitate the need for research.

UNDERSTANDING THE NEEDS OF THE COMMUNITY: THE DISASTER PSYCHOSOCIAL ASSESSMENT AND SURVEILLANCE TOOLKIT (DISASTER-PAST)

Anthony Speier, associate professor at the Louisiana State University Health Sciences Center, described the Disaster Psychosocial Assessment and Surveillance Toolkit (Disaster-PAST), developed to better understand the "who, what, where, when, and how" of recovering communities through surveillance of community mental health and psychosocial functioning following disasters.[2] Tracking basic demographic information, such as where people are living before a disaster, can help in planning for where services will be needed when people start returning after being displaced by the disaster. He concurred with Bradberry that disasters are highly politicized, and it helps to have a more quantitative and objective method of assessing where the needs are, and what services should be added to address those needs.

Data-informed knowledge helps determine what level of service is needed and allows funding sources to direct an appropriate level of services to those needs, Speier said. Disaster-PAST can also help to identify which populations are most in need of mental health services after a disaster and can identify risk factors for developing certain types

---

[2]The toolkit was designed for use by any agency or entity and is free and publicly available. See http://www.medschool.lsuhsc.edu/psychiatry/disasterpast_contents.aspx (accessed November 10, 2014).

of mental illness following a disaster. The toolkit also provides recommendations of when to conduct the assessment and surveillance following a disaster, including guidance for ongoing evaluation and long-term surveillance of mental health needs over time. The main purpose of the toolkit is to provide guidance on how to conduct psychosocial surveillance after a disaster (e.g., screening tools, sampling) and how to use that information to inform provision of services to help the community.

Speier concluded by highlighting the key elements of preparing a community for participation in disaster impact research, such as Disaster-PAST, that overlapped with key points from previous speakers. He recommended the following:

- A prearranged community research advisory board strategy (e.g., knowing who the stakeholders are and how those people can be encouraged to become involved in the research design and data gathering);
- Observable, tangible actions to foster community trust (e.g., following through on promises made to the community);
- An easily understood script regarding direct benefits of the research for the community; and
- Clinical support for participants embedded within the research design and data gathering.

CHALLENGES AND OPPORTUNITIES

A recurring theme throughout the community discussion was the need to reach out and partner with other groups and establish trusting relationships and grassroots connections among public health, academia, and all appropriate community stakeholders before the disaster, which Herrmann summarized in his report of the panel session (see Box 5-1). A challenge is identifying the "right" partners and finding the resources and mechanisms to develop and maintain these relationships, as academic institutions, are not funded for relationship building.

A suggestion was made that local and state health departments especially need to be engaged as partners before a disaster, as they are often overwhelmed during the response and bombarded with requests. With regard to funding predisaster research and relationship building, it

BOX 5-1
Partnering with the Community to Enable Research[a]

Challenges and Issues

- How to establish trust with the community predisaster
- Lack of preexisting relationships among public health, academia, and other important stakeholders
- Lack of clarity of research benefit to the community
- "You only care about us in a disaster"

Opportunities for Improvement

- Preestablished partnership agreements between public health and academia
- Early involvement and engagement of the community in research planning; research that improves recovery should be a key part of planning
- Work with health educators and others to translate research data for community understanding
- Work with academic researchers and clinicians who are already working with the community on a day-to-day basis

Critical Partnerships and Collaborations

- Health departments
- The "mayors" of the community, community-based organizations, faith-based organizations
- Local universities and colleges
- Politicos

[a]The challenges, opportunities, and partnerships listed were identified by one or more individual participants in this breakout panel discussion. This summary was prepared by the panel facilitator and presented in the subsequent plenary session. This list is not meant to reflect a consensus among workshop participants.

SOURCE: Plenary session summary of breakout panel discussion as reported by panel facilitator Jack Herrmann.

was noted that local health departments often have internships for students in public health programs. How can the resources of universities be leveraged to help the health department gather data prior to an event?

It was also noted that many local health departments are working toward accreditation by the Public Health Accreditation Board, and among the measures are building partnerships, working with students, and being involved in research. Participants also noted the need to identify the unofficial "mayors," the people who are recognized as leaders within the community, Herrmann summarized. Additionally, there is a lack of clarity around the benefit of conducting research in the community, Herrmann explained. A participant noted the value of risk communication in helping people who are emotionally stressed to understand how the research affects them and the health of their community without inundating them with data, as Bradberry mentioned previously.

> Y'all come to our region when disasters come. Nobody comes when we're talking about enhancing the infrastructure, the capacity beforehand. We're the poorest, have the most health needs, and the only time you come is when we have a disaster.
>
> —*Participant from Mississippi*

A participant said there is an opportunity to work with first responder organizations, community leaders, and others to find the commonalities across the country and start thinking about "plug and play" protocols. Participants discussed balancing respect for the diversity and distinct cult-ures of communities with the development of standardized, ready-made research protocols. Additionally, further concerns were raised about researchers who impose their own ideas on a community, rather than take the time to understand what the community needs, and the impact of the onslaught of researchers into a community after a disaster. A participant said that people descend into the Gulf region when disasters happen, but nobody comes when the region is talking about enhancing the infrastructure and the capacity beforehand. The region is the poorest and has the most health needs, but the only time researchers come is when there is a disaster, they said.

6

Improving Data Collection Capabilities and Information Resources

Simply collecting data in disasters often presents its own set of barriers. Sometimes the data just do not exist, or tools to collect information have to be recreated or are too clunky for mobile research studies, or curated databases are not made available to open audiences. To address pieces of this, data collection could often be legitimately framed as disaster epidemiology, with an expected impact on public health practice, which may remove some of the administrative challenges often encountered. In this section, participants explored new data collection tools, strategies, and infrastructure needs across many sectors to enable effective and accessible data sharing and field implementation.

To open the discussion on data collection, Steven Phillips, associate director of NLM, shared several examples of information field tools developed by the NLM Disaster Information Management Research Center and in use in disasters. He described a few quick tools they have been tracking that would assist research responders, sometimes in austere environments, in data collection. One is a digital pen that writes like a regular pen but also stores the information that is written (e.g., on a triage form) and sends the information to wherever it needs to be (e.g., the hospital). Another example is a "lost person finder" that simply uses a smart phone camera as a tool to upload photos to an online bulletin board so family and friends can locate each other. Radiofrequency identification tags are used to track patients, equipment, and tools. Responder guidance tools and disaster-related apps are also available to assist first responders, such as the Wireless Information System for Emergency

Responders, Radiation Emergency Medical Management, and Chemical Hazards Emergency Medical Management.[1]

NIH DISASTER RESEARCH RESPONSE PROJECT

Aubrey Miller, senior medical advisor at NIEHS, expanded on the DR2 project discussed previously by Birnbaum. He reiterated that the project was initiated by NIEHS and NLM to help address the slow deployment of research that leads to the loss of perishable data. Creating a central repository of standardized tools and developing easy-to-use preset protocols for researchers to use during disasters are two main priorities as this project continues to develop. This standardization of tools and protocols will assist both the research teams conducting the study as well as the communities where the research is being performed so they do not have to adapt to new technologies and systems each time a new team wants to collect data.

The first part of the DR2 project is the creation of a central repository of publicly available data collection tools that could be used to help establish early baselines and cohorts for research. Such tools could include surveys, questionnaires, implementation guidance, forms (e.g., clinical testing, consent), and research protocols. Following a comprehensive search, more than 400 of the research tools identified were chosen for evaluation, Miller said, and about 200 were selected for initial inclusion in the database. The repository, housed on the NLM Disaster Research Responder website, is intended to be an easy-to-use, interactive site where researchers can find tools to support research response. The searchable repository will also include metadata about the tools (e.g., ease of use, duration, number of questions, languages the tool is available in, history of use, points of contact for the tool, references, etc.). Ultimately, there could be "drag and drop" type functionality to create new tools specific to a researcher's needs and have validation. Miller also noted the intent to have preapproval by the NIEHS IRB and the Office of Management and Budget (OMB), to the extent possible, for use of some of the low-impact research tools (e.g., tools to measure respiratory impacts or eye, ear, nose, or throat irritation).

Another aspect of the project is developing the capacity for rapid data collection. NIEHS is working on how to deploy intramural clinical

---

[1]For more information on all of these tools, see http://disaster.nlm.nih.gov/dimrc/tools nlmdimrc.html (accessed November 3, 2014).

program assets, with support from contracting capabilities, to collect baseline and early data (e.g., questionnaire information, biospecimens, perhaps environmental samples). Part of this rapid data collection capability is the development of a "plug and play" research protocol, Miller explained, that would have preexisting IRB approvals and that could then be sent back through the IRB for a quick approval.

One of the next steps in the DR2 project is engaging a broad array of NIH intramural and extramural researchers, stakeholders, and consortia in an environmental health science "research response network." This national network would help develop and prioritize tools and training materials, help to evaluate and improve research response concepts, and foster wider participation among the environmental health community (including citizen scientists). Other ongoing activities include training and exercising the tools and implementation plans (e.g., the tabletop exercise conducted in Los Angeles).

DISASTER EPIDEMIOLOGY: APPLIED PUBLIC HEALTH INVESTIGATION AND RESEARCH DURING DISASTERS

Michael Heumann of Heumann Health Consulting and a consultant for the Council of State and Territorial Epidemiologists (CSTE) provided an overview of disaster epidemiology and shared examples of how a variety of standard epidemiological methods are being applied in the public health response to disasters and disaster research (see Figure 6-1).

Heumann defined disaster epidemiology as applying the tools of epidemiology to assess short- and long-term health effects of disasters, and to predict the consequences for future disasters. It is an applied public health practice that is closely linked to disaster research. The goals of disaster epidemiology are to prevent or reduce deaths, illness, and injuries caused by disasters and to provide timely and accurate health information for decision makers. Heumann suggested that disaster epidemiologists should be research partners and providers of some of the baseline data that disaster researchers seek. Aligning public health practice and research will be important as disaster epidemiology becomes more common, and stronger partnerships can help both medical and public health responders and researchers achieve their goals. Disaster

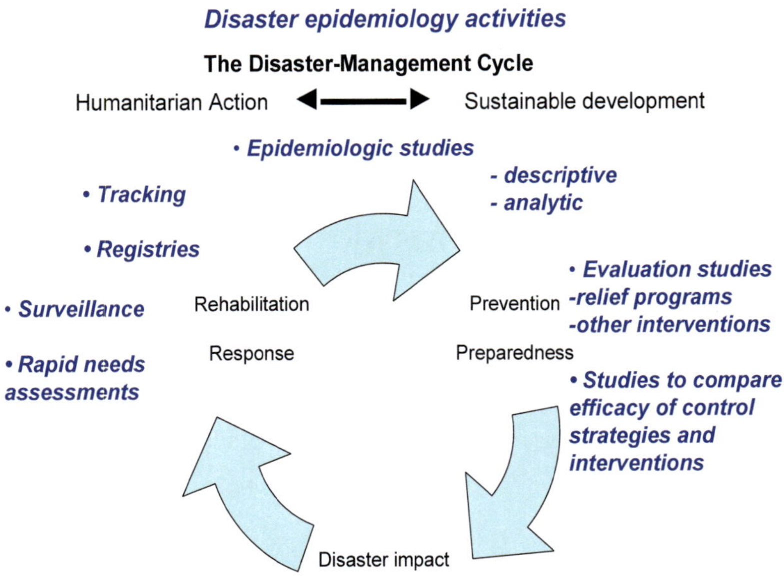

FIGURE 6-1 Disaster epidemiology conceptual framework describing the applications of epidemiology in the disaster management cycle developed by the Council of State and Territorial Epidemiologists in collaboration with the National Center for Environmental Health at the Centers for Disease Control and Prevention.
SOURCE: Heumann presentation, June 13, 2014.

epidemiology also seeks to improve prevention and mitigation strategies for future disasters by gaining information for response preparation.

Disaster epidemiologists face a variety of challenges during a disaster, many of which are related to collecting data. There is often an absence of baseline information, denominator data are difficult to obtain, electronic health data might be limited and medical or death records might not indicate disaster-relatedness. Infrastructure damage (e.g., power, phone, and Internet outages), logistical constraints (e.g., environmental hazards, blocked roads, fuel shortages), and competing priorities also impact disaster epidemiology.

Heumann stressed the importance of integrating disaster epidemiology and accompanying research across disciplines (e.g., acute diseases, chronic diseases, communicable diseases, environmental and occupational health, injury assessment) and collaborating with partners in public health, hospitals, academic partners, industrial hygiene and safety professionals, emergency managers, responders, volunteer organizations, and the community.

Disaster Epidemiology Resources

As a partner discipline, disaster epidemiology has a variety of resources to offer. Heumann gave an example from a recent disaster for each type of resource:

- Rapid needs assessments (e.g., assessment of community public health needs after a massive Texas wildfire).
- Shelter surveillance (e.g., for shelters set up after Hurricane Sandy, monitored for outbreaks, illnesses, exacerbations of chronic conditions).
- Morbidity and mortality surveillance (e.g., tracking in Moore, Oklahoma, after 2013 tornadoes).
- Responder health and safety surveillance (e.g., roster and track >55,000 workers during Gulf oil spill and response).
- Descriptive and analytic studies (e.g., description of injuries and fatalities resulting from fertilizer plant explosion in West, Texas).
- Evaluation and impact studies (e.g., evaluation of long-term community recovery after Hurricane Andrew).
- Registries (e.g., post-9/11 WTC registry created to monitor health effects of survivors).

Heumann highlighted three specific examples of disaster epidemiology resources, all of which were developed by CDC and could be mobilized quickly after a disaster if needed. CASPER[2] is an epidemiological technique designed to provide rapid and low-cost, household-based information about community needs in a simple format for decision makers. The CASPER methodology involves a two-stage probability sample using 30 clusters based on Census blocks and randomly choosing seven households per block to participate in a household-level interview. Data are then weighted to adjust for non-

[2]Also discussed by Lakey in the panel discussion on Partnering with the Community to Enable Access and Baseline Data.

random sampling, and statistically relevant population-based estimates are obtained. Heumann noted that reports are generated within about 72 hours of data collection and shared with partners (including the community where the data were obtained).

ERHMS[3] is a health monitoring and surveillance framework for protecting responders through all phases of a response. Heumann noted that the work done in the predeployment phase is similar to the work already being done by fire departments, hazmat teams, and EMS units in terms of training and credentialing, although the documentation is different. ERHMS data are entered into a larger database that is part of the deployment database. Thus, the ERHMS system can track and roster responders during the deployment phase and conduct surveillance and monitoring for exposures and health effects. All of this information is analyzed in the postdeployment phase, which also includes follow-up with responders about their experiences, referral for additional follow-up as needed, or enrollment into medium- or long-term surveillance for delayed adverse effects.

The Assessment of Chemical Exposures program, developed by the Agency for Toxic Substances and Disease Registry, provides training in disaster epidemiological investigation of a chemical incident, technical assistance, and a toolkit of resources to guide local authorities in response. The toolkit includes standardized materials, such as modifiable survey forms, consent forms, a medical chart abstraction form, an interviewer training manual, and databases.[4]

Disaster epidemiology is now widely practiced, Heumann said, and most local and state health departments carry out some form of disaster epidemiology. CDC deploys field teams, on request from local and state health departments, to provide technical assistance or to lead a response activity in major incidents. The need now is to develop stronger linkages and alignment between public health practice and research. A critical aspect of disaster epidemiology response and research is partnerships, Heumann said. In particular, public health has to be part of the ICS. Disaster epidemiology is a core tool that public health brings to the table, he said. There must also be integration of local, state, and federal engagement. Other key partnerships are between health departments and academia, between applied public health (including epidemiology) and research, and between disaster epidemiology and social science research. Heumann noted that disaster epidemiology data collection does not

---

[3]Discussed by Howard in the plenary session (see Chapter 2).

[4]See http://www.atsdr.cdc.gov/ntsip/ace.html (accessed September 30, 2014).

require IRB approval, and a key factor in making the data useful for researchers is deidentification and anonymization.

THE NATIONAL EMERGENCY MEDICAL SERVICES INFORMATION SYSTEM

Gamunu Wijetunge and Ellen Schenk of the Office of Emergency Medical Services at the National Highway Traffic Safety Administration (NHTSA) provided a brief overview of the federal role in supporting the development of EMS and described NEMSIS and its role in supporting preparedness planning and research.

NEMSIS

NEMSIS is a system for standardizing EMS patient care data collection across the United States by promoting the use of standard definitions, data formats, and data reporting, Wijetunge explained. NEMSIS currently includes standard definitions and formats for more than 400 data elements (version 2). When emergency medical technicians (EMTs) and paramedics treat a patient at the scene of an incident, information about the incident and the care provided is documented on an electronic patient care report (EPCR). The data elements in that EPCR come from the standardized NEMSIS dataset. There are 83 specific national elements within the larger national dataset that are reported to the NEMSIS Technical Assistance Center, housed at the University of Utah, to populate the National EMS Database. In addition, states and localities select additional elements to collect to stay at the state and local level based on their data needs. Wijetunge noted that 47 states and territories currently submit NEMSIS-compliant data describing EMS events to the National EMS Database, which now contains more than 30 million patient care records.

Using NEMSIS in Research

Schenk presented several examples of how NEMSIS could be used to conduct research and obtain information during disasters. EMS dispatch data in NEMSIS could be used to monitor requests for emergency services realtime during a disaster (e.g., during major flooding) and to prepare the emergency response for similar disasters in other areas. During the 2009 H1N1 pandemic, NEMSIS data showed the number of people in Florida reporting that they were sick to an EMS dispatcher. A statistically significant temporal pattern was observed, Schenk said, and Florida public health officials could watch this information in real time and respond to the event. Other geographic areas with similar demographics to Florida (particularly with a large percentage of the population at high risk for flu) could learn from the trends in Florida to prepare for responses to future flu pandemics.

In a more detailed example, Schenk and colleagues used data from the NEMSIS National EMS Database to characterize and estimate the frequency of mass casualty incidents (MCIs) occurring in the United States in 2010, as reported by EMS personnel (Schenk et al., 2014). Of the roughly 9.8 million EMS responses in the 2010 database, 14,504 (0.15 percent) were recorded as MCIs. Among these entries, it was estimated that there were nearly 10,000 unique incidents and 14,000 unique patients, which translated to an observed rate of 13 MCIs per 100,000 population and 1.7 MCIs per 1,000 calls to 911. Overall, Schenk said, the study found that MCIs are smaller in scale and more frequent in nature than expected and that response delays were reported to be more common for MCI EMS responses than for non-MCI responses. Schenk is conducting further research on factors that could explain the response delay, as well as looking into perceptions of EMS personnel regarding a response being an MCI. She noted that the study also shows some of the limitations of the current infrastructure of NEMSIS for providing information on disasters. Not all patients involved in a particular MCI may be documented, because some state and local EMS systems have protocols that permit EMS personnel to reduce the time devoted to patient documentation and tracking during larger, more complex incidents. Thus, NEMSIS currently provides fairly accurate information on trends and percentages as well as the count of events, but not the absolute count of patients. Another limitation is that NEMSIS is not currently a population-based, or nationally representative, sample, but this improves every day as more states and more agencies submit their data to the national level, Schenk said. Also, the subjectivity of the NEMSIS definition of MCI provides both opportunities and challenges for conducting research.

In closing, Schenk encouraged participants to consider EMS as a valuable source of data for conducting research and obtaining information during and after disasters and to explore NEMSIS for utility in their preparedness planning and research efforts.[5] NEMSIS can mitigate some of the common challenges of conducting disaster research by providing baseline information, the capacity to conduct longitudinal health assessments for high-risk groups, and deidentified data.

DISASTER RESEARCH AND RESPONSE: APPLIED PUBLIC HEALTH PERSPECTIVE

CDC's National Center for Environmental Health (NCEH) is the lead CDC center in responses to natural, chemical, and radiological disasters. The Office of Public Health Preparedness and Response provides overall coordination and support of CDC activities and funds state and local capacity building efforts, and the Center for Surveillance, Epidemiology, and Laboratory Services houses the BioSense public health surveillance system.[6]

The Health Studies Branch of NCEH focuses on building public health capacity at the state and local levels, providing assistance and emergency response during events, and conducting research on risk and protective factors, said Lauren Lewis, chief of the Health Studies Branch at NCEH. The center obtains data in the course of providing technical assistance to its partners, including state and local public health offices and nongovernmental organizations (NGOs), for the primary purpose of public health decision making. NCEH publishes much of the data that are collected in the course of providing a service to facilitate additional research.

Lewis provided several examples of how data collected by NCEH inform public health. For example, NCEH conducted mental health assessments following the Deepwater Horizon oil spill and identified a need for increased mental health services in the region. Using that data, impacted states were then able to obtain funding from BP to increase mental health services. Following the tsunami in American Samoa, NCEH assisted with clinical surveillance and was able to identify injuries as a priority. In addition, surveillance did not detect outbreaks of infectious diseases, and this information was used to combat rumors, Lewis said.

---

[5]See http://nemsis.org (accessed June 12, 2014).
[6]See http://www.cdc.gov/biosense (accessed June 12, 2014).

Coordinating Across Organizations for Surveillance

NCEH works closely with the American Red Cross and has developed standardized morbidity and mortality data collection tools for the Red Cross volunteers to use in the course of their activities. Data collected are sent to CDC for analysis and are reported back to the Red Cross in the form of information they can use. For example, NCEH worked with the American Red Cross during the Alabama tornadoes in 2011. Workers collected standardized information when they provided services to families of decedents, and NCEH analyzed the circumstances surrounding the fatalities. Women and the elderly were identified as the highest risk groups, and most people died in single-family homes, unexpected findings that have generated much discussion, Lewis noted.

NCEH also partners with the American Association of Poison Control Centers and conducts surveillance of the National Poison Data System. NCEH monitors calls to all 57 U.S. poison centers and receives alerts when there are anomalies in the data that might indicate an event of public health significance. This tool is used in nearly every disaster, Lewis said. For example, NCEH tracks carbon monoxide poisonings during disasters that result in power outages. The system is also used to monitor public concerns and push information out to the public. During the Fukushima meltdown, there was a rise in calls related to iodine poisonings, and NCEH realized that people were taking iodine out of fear. In response, CDC issued communication to educate the public.

Future Directions

Response data make very good data for evaluating programs, Lewis said. Response data are useful for comparison in future studies (e.g., initial versus 1-year follow-up) and for generating hypotheses and designing research studies (e.g., high-risk groups that should be tracked). Data collected for public health practice, such as FEMA claims data, do have identifiable information, Lewis noted, and potentially could be used to identify participants for future research. Lewis concurred with some of the challenges of disaster research mentioned by others, including issues related to the IRBs, OMB, and funding for response versus research.

NCEH is now focusing on improving the data collected during a response, not only for immediate public health actions, but also for research. There is interest in an electronic death registry system and how to link death records to an event for disaster mortality surveillance. There is also interest in using social media to track disaster-related deaths (e.g., online memorial sites, blogs), although the information posted is generally not very specific. NCEH is also working with emergency managers on institutionalizing the use of data from research, particularly social vulnerability tools and information.

CHALLENGES AND OPPORTUNITIES

A key issue highlighted in the panel discussions is the need for common infrastructure of terminology and definitions, data collecting, reporting of information, and broad dissemination, Steven Phillips reported in his summary of the session (see Box 6-1). The need for a central repository of data was also discussed, as well as a centralized list (website) of data collection and reporting tools.

A participant raised the issue of actually collecting disaster epidemiology data. While the guidance, tools, and standardized templates are helpful, many rural counties have very small health departments and simply do not have the staff to be in the field collecting data. Heumann noted that sometimes the state has expectations of what localities can provide, and there needs to be dialogue or negotiation about how localities can meet those expectations with the resources they have. There is training available in Disaster Epidemiology through the Health Studies Branch of CDC,[7] including in-person, long-distance, webinar, and self-study modules. Miller added that in the face of shrinking resources, the federal government can only do so much, and it is time to engage a much broader community to participate in gathering information (e.g., academia, NGOs, community groups).

A participant suggested selecting some sites where disasters are predicted to happen as test areas to validate collecting baseline data before an event (e.g., floods in the Midwest, hurricanes in the East, wildfires in Southern California or Texas). Heumann concurred, adding that much of the data of interest probably already exist, for example, in electronic health records and other systems, the task is to figure out how to harness those data. Lewis noted that the Environmental Health Tracking Network does have the potential to provide baseline data.

---

[7]See http://www.cdc.gov/nceh/hsb/disaster/training.htm (accessed November 10, 2014)

BOX 6-1
Improving Data Collection Capabilities and Information Resources[a]

Challenges and Issues

- Common terminology, definitions, and collection and reporting systems
- Central repository for data (bidirectional)
- Research goals include helping victim outcomes
- Creating partnership between disparate agencies/groups with a common mission; integrate existing networks

Opportunities for Improvement

- List (website) of collection and reporting tools
- Determine "what is out there" that works or might work
- Collect and provide predisaster health information on responders and victims (a universal electronic health record)

Critical Partnerships and Collaborations

- Local, state, regional, and national agencies, with Congress, to enact consensus legislation
- Communities, clubs, nongovernmental organizations, and agencies
- Who pays? (Centers for Medicare & Medicaid Services, private insurers, other partners?)

[a]The challenges, opportunities, and partnerships listed were identified by one or more individual participants in this breakout panel discussion. This summary was prepared by the panel facilitator and presented in the subsequent plenary session. This list is not meant to reflect a consensus among workshop participants.

SOURCE: Plenary session summary of breakout panel discussion as reported by panel facilitator Steven Phillips.

Another common theme throughout the presentations was partnerships, and panelists gave more details on their own experiences. One of the challenges, Heumann said, is that partners may feel they have proprietary ownership of their information, and they have concerns about how others might use it. Developing relationships and trust is the key to understanding and to developing cooperation, he said. Shared goals and objectives, and respect for each other's boundaries, have to be established and agreed to, sometimes in writing. Steven Phillips said that standards in terminology, data collection, and data reporting could help to eliminate the silos and the territorial boundaries and make partnerships easier to develop, like what is being done through NEMSIS. Miller reiterated the importance of laying the groundwork and connecting with people, helping people to understand that the government is there to help. A partnership has to be mutually beneficial, Lewis said. Often, the research we want to do is not aligned with the missions and priorities of the partners that we need to help collect the data (e.g., clinicians, state and local public health). Clinicians can ask a few extra questions during care to collect data, but how can that also help them in their mission? Wijetunge reiterated the importance of personal relationships with staff at other agencies. Schenk added that the first step is sharing information and getting people to talk to each other. A few involved participants also highlighted that the goal of collecting data is to improve victim outcomes. This involves engaging the affected populations to understand their needs and helping them to understand why collecting this information is important. A question raised by participants was who ultimately pays for improving data collection infrastructure (e.g., CMS, private insurers, other partners), a topic that will be discussed at greater length in the next chapter.

7

Considerations for Rapid and Sustained Funding Mechanisms for Research in Disasters

This section focused on rapid funding mechanisms that could enable nimble and flexible grant distribution. Participants discussed strategies for designing funding mechanisms that would allow for sustainable disaster research protocols and that have the flexibility to immediately activate additional protocols during a disaster. Gwen Collman, director of the Division of Extramural Research and Training at NIH, highlighted several of the NIEHS options for funding of extramural research on disasters. The NIEHS Mechanism for Time-Sensitive Research Opportunities in Environmental Health Sciences (R21), for example, funds the collection of data when there is an unforeseen opportunity that requires rapid mobilization, establishment of a study population, and specimen collection. Another mechanism is funding through the network of NIH Centers of Excellence. Each NIH center has some discretion to move money quickly for pilot projects that meet center mandates. Centers can ask for rebudgeting of funds that are already in their core budgets or use their own pilot project fund. Additional nonfederal mechanisms and sources of funding are also discussed that could potentially be used for quick disbursement and research.

NSF RAPID AWARDS

Dennis Wenger, program director for the Infrastructure Systems Management and Extreme Events program at NSF, described the NSF Grants for Rapid Response Research program (referred to as RAPID awards). According to NSF, "the RAPID funding mechanism is used for proposals having a severe urgency with regard to availability of, or access to, data, facilities, or specialized equipment, including quick-response research on natural and anthropogenic disasters and similar unanticipated events."[1] Importantly, NSF also has a very well-organized extramural research community of disaster-science social scientists.

Proposals for RAPID are brief (two to five pages) and must include a clear description of why the proposed research is of an urgent nature and why a RAPID award would be the most appropriate funding mechanism. Before submitting a RAPID proposal, investigators must first contact the individual program officer whose expertise is closest to the proposed topic to determine whether the proposed work is appropriate for RAPID funding, Wenger explained. RAPID proposals are subject to internal merit review, and the funding decision resides with the program officer. Awards are up to $200,000 for 1 year and typically take only 1 or 2 weeks to process and award funding. Program officers are also allowed to make a decision of up to $50,000 without undergoing external peer review, giving them even greater flexibility and shortening time lines to just a few days. In contrast, the R21 mechanism Collman described from NIEHS is poised to release funding 3 months after submission at the earliest.[2] However, Farris Tuma, from the National Institute of Mental Health (NIMH) at NIH, noted that within NIMH the R21 funding opportunities titled, "Rapid Assessment Post-Impact of Disaster" take approximately 8 weeks from submission to award. This includes initial peer review, second-level council review, and processing by the grants office. Once an application has been reviewed and recommended for funding, the money can flow in days. Wenger added that because NSF RAPID awards do not undergo the same rigorous external peer-review process associated with unsolicited proposals and career proposals, program officers may not spend more than a total of 5 percent of their annual budget on RAPID awards (there is no annual budget for RAPID awards).

In most cases, RAPID awards result from investigators approaching NSF about a potential proposal. In some cases, however, program officers draft a Dear Colleague Letter that is sent out broadly to the research community, calling for RAPID proposals. The Dear Colleague Letter is generally used during a major disaster, and there is usually a short deadline

---

[1]See http://www.nsf.gov/pubs/policydocs/pappguide/nsf09_1/gpg_2.jsp#IID1, D. Special Guidelines, 1. Grants for Rapid Response Research (RAPID) (accessed December 16, 2014).

[2]For more on the Mechanism for Time-Sensitive Research Opportunities in Environmental Health Sciences, see http://grants.nih.gov/grants/guide/pa-files/PAR-13-136.html (accessed December 16, 2014).

for proposals (2 weeks). This approach to call for proposals was used, for example, after Hurricanes Katrina and Sandy, the Indian Ocean tsunami, the earthquakes in Haiti and New Zealand, and the Fukushima nuclear disaster. As an example, Wenger said that after Hurricane Katrina, NSF received 170 inquiries about RAPID awards, 134 draft proposals were submitted, 80 were then submitted as RAPID proposals, and about 50 awards were made within 3 weeks.

Wenger said that in addition to the RAPID awards, NSF supports other initiatives that support quick response research. The Earthquake Engineering Research Institute (EERI), for example, has the Learning from Earthquakes program that is supported by NSF, and allows multi-disciplinary teams of engineers, geoscientists, social scientists, and others to rapidly get on-site after an earthquake (although there is currently no health component to this program). The Natural Hazard Center at the University of Colorado, funded by NSF and other federal agencies, has a quick response program. At the beginning of the year, researchers submit brief proposals, and if an event occurs during the year that is related to a qualified proposal, funding would be approved (generally small grants of about $5,000 to assist with data collection). If the hazard or situation in the proposal does not occur during that year, researchers can apply again the next year.

PRIVATE FUNDING: GRANTMAKERS IN HEALTH

Grantmakers In Health is the professional association for health foundations and corporate donors, said President and CEO Faith Mitchell.[3] Association membership includes hundreds of foundations and other funding partners. Many health foundations are local, Mitchell explained. Many grew out of local nonprofit organizations, some were started by families, and some came about as a result of the conversion when a non-profit health provider was sold to a for-profit hospital or other institution (by law, the proceeds of the sale are to be used for charitable purposes in the same area that was served by the nonprofit organization). About half of the members of Grantmakers In Health are local funders, about one-quarter are state based, and about one-quarter are national. They range from small to huge, Mitchell said. The Colorado Health Foundation, for example, provides grants to improve health and health care in Colorado and has more than $2 billion in assets.

---

[3]See http://www.gih.org (accessed December 16, 2014).

Many of the association members are involved in disaster-related work, primarily related to response and recovery. Local foundations often see their role as serving the local community, and there is a lot of interest in community rebuilding. Many of the state and local foundations have emergency grantmaking procedures in place to provide rapid funding to organizations that are serving the immediate needs of residents in their communities. Larger foundations such as Robert Wood Johnson Foundation and others have a general interest in preparedness and often fund health-related research. Foundations also have the ability to write checks very quickly if they have to, Mitchell said, certainly more quickly than the typical government agency.

Membership Foundations

Mitchell shared several examples of ongoing work by member foundations. The New York Community Trust has been making grants to continue rebuilding neighborhoods that were hit by Hurricane Sandy. In addition to rebuilding the infrastructure of New York City, they are also using their funding to develop a disaster preparedness and response plan for elderly New Yorkers and to help protect recovery workers from injury through hazardous conditions. They also provided online legal resources for people affected by the storm and provided grant support to manage a community planning process for affected neighborhoods. The Conrad Hilton Foundation, based in California, is a national and international funder that supports immediate and longer-term assistance for people affected by natural disasters and promotes disaster preparedness. Through their Responding to National Disasters program, it awarded Harvard University $400,000 to scale up the Harvard Humanitarian Initiatives KoBo toolbox application suite. This toolbox application was designed to improve the coordination and evaluation of disaster response efforts and allows for on-the-ground, handheld, digital data collection. Another initiative is the Rockefeller Foundation's 100 Resilient Cities Centennial Challenge. This is a $100 million commitment to provide grants to 100 cities around the world to address preparedness planning, including meeting the needs of vulnerable residents during a response. The 100 cities that receive grants also receive technical assistance and support in creating and implementing their plans, membership into a learning network of all the grantee cities, and support for hiring a chief resilience officer who will oversee the development of a resilience plan for their city. Thirty-two cities have already been selected.

In summary, Mitchell said, private foundations can move quickly, have a strong community-orientation focus, and are generally interested in applied response and recovery activities, rather than research, but there is an emerging interest in research that is directed to solving community needs.

OTHER FEDERAL FUNDING

Sarah A. Lister, specialist in public health and epidemiology at the Congressional Research Service (CRS),[4] described some of the options available for funding disaster response, and the health aspects of response, from a congressional point of view. As background, Lister explained that the Anti-Deficiency Act essentially says that the federal government cannot spend money that has not been provided to it in advance through appropriations or other congressional action. There is, however, an exception that allows the government to accept volunteer services in order to preserve life and property in an emergency.[5]

Some specific mechanisms allow for spending on disaster response. Ideally, there would be an existing fund that is preserved until needed in emergency and disbursed only under certain conditions. There are few examples of this in the federal government. There is authority in the Public Health Service Act for the HHS Secretary to have a rainy day fund that she can access if she declares a public health emergency; however, there is no money in that fund. Although Congress did put in money in the late 1990s to be used for Y2K-related problems, Lister said it has never put money in the fund to be available for "as yet undetermined" purposes. A more realistic example is the Disaster Relief Fund administered by FEMA under the Stafford Act. When the president, at the request of one or more governors, declares that a major disaster or emergency exists (a Stafford Act declaration), FEMA can task other federal agencies with Mission Assignments, which are activities that are not already funded through their own budgets but for which they will be reimbursed from the Disaster Relief Fund. FEMA regulations for implementing the Stafford Act and providing

---

[4]CRS provides direct policy analysis and support exclusively to Congress. Although CRS reports may be in circulation, CRS does not have a public mission or a public website where the public can access reports. CRS provides authoritative expertise and analysis that is non-partisan and neutral. CRS does not make recommendations, but does present analyses of viable options.

[5]Section 1342 of Title 31 of the U.S. Code can be accessed at http://www.gpo.gov/fdsys/pkg/USCODE-2011-title31/html/USCODE-2011-title31-subtitleII-chap13-subchapIII-sec1342.htm (accessed on November 10, 2014).

assistance do not explicitly address whether "ephemeral disaster research" can be justified as essential or nonessential, and arguments could be made either way, Lister added. Continuing to work with ASPR to develop clearer taxonomy related to disaster research response could be a useful path forward to aid in securing this type of funding.

Although the Stafford Act does not preclude an emergency declaration for a principally health event, Lister noted that there is only one example of using the Disaster Relief Fund for a chemical, biological, or radiological incident with a health component that did not also involve the destruction of infrastructure. This was an emergency declaration made in the response to the introduction of West Nile virus into the United States in the late 1990s. The Disaster Relief Fund was used for FEMA Mission Assignments allowing CDC and other HHS agencies to provide assistance to New York, Connecticut, and other states with outbreaks. The Disaster Relief Fund was not used for the flu pandemic in 2009. The bulk of that response, Lister said, was funded through supplemental appropriation from Congress, which was enacted about 2 months after the HHS Secretary declared the emergency.[6]

Transfer Authority and Budgets

The HHS Secretary and the directors of HHS agencies also have a certain amount of standing transfer authority. In their annual appropriations, Congress grants them the ability to move a small percentage of money around for uses other than the explicit allocations that Congress has provided. This transfer authority is used often, Lister said. The Secretary used it, for example, to fund implementation of the Affordable Care Act and the health care exchanges in 2013. The transfer authority is not limited to any particular purpose and could be used in an emergency if money is available, she suggested. She added that the further an agency is into the fiscal year, the less money there is available to move around for these purposes (i.e., they simply may not have 2 percent of their annual budget left in unobligated funds as they near the end of the summer).[7] For example, the Substance Abuse and Mental Health Services Administration has a 3 percent reprogramming authority for disasters. However, if a new budget is not passed and continuing resolutions run for several months beyond

---

[6]For the full text of the Supplemental Appropriations Act, 2009, Public Law No. 111-32, 123 Stat. 1884-1886, see http://www.gpo.gov/fdsys/pkg/PLAW-111publ32/pdf/PLAW-111publ32.pdf (accessed December 16, 2014).

[7]The U.S. federal government's fiscal year is October 1 through September 30.

October 1, the agency may have no new funding to reprogram during hurricane season.

More flexibility is built into some agencies' budgets. For example, the U.S. Food and Drug Administration (FDA) anticipates that some of its inspection resources are going to be deployed in an unanticipated manner (e.g., for inspections related to food-borne illness outbreaks), but it does not have much flexibility in its ability to do unanticipated intramural research. The CDC budget builds in flexibility to provide assistance to states and other public health entities for unanticipated events, and there is some flexibility in its ability to do unanticipated intramural research, but less so for grant making. Funding from private foundations can be used to support agency actions directly only with the permission of Congress, Lister explained. CDC, for example, has a congressionally chartered foundation with an emergency fund. Supplemental appropriations are used by Congress to address health emergencies for which assistance under the Stafford Act is insufficient or unavailable, or when inherent flexibility, transfer authorities, foundation funding, or other mechanisms fall short. However, Lister reiterated that supplemental appropriations from Congress can take some time.

In general, Lister said, there are often difficulties in finding ways to fund the health response to a disaster. In many cases, agencies would like to act, but they do not have a clear source of payment to cover their actions, or if they do have funds available, they are not necessarily available legally. It would be ideal if responders at the federal level could have more certainty about where funds might come from for immediate research that might be needed in a disaster. Lister noted that in a resource-constrained environment, Congress has been reluctant to fund the secretary's Public Health Emergency Fund. There has also been discussion in the homeland security and disaster preparedness communities about whether it works well for the Disaster Relief Fund to be the central pot of money for all disasters, or whether each department should have its own version of a disaster relief fund. In closing, Lister noted that what is considered an emergency in terms of research may vary. For example, applied public health research, such as characterizing a new virus or developing a new laboratory test, may be "an easy sell," while establishing a registry of exposure during an incident is a tougher sell, as this is not really research but setting the stage for future research.

CHALLENGES AND OPPORTUNITIES

As reported by Gwen Collman in her summary (see Box 7-1), some participants discussed issues surrounding the time it takes to award funding to investigators, the size of the awards, statutory issues related to the funding source, and the time frame to complete the research. With regard to access to funding, a participant suggested that the vast majority of people who are doing disaster research are not aware of the various funding opportunities described by the panelists. In addition, rapid response funding is disproportionately shifted toward infrastructure and engineering, as opposed to the full dimensions of human health. In this regard, some participants noted the need to raise awareness about the health aspects of disasters and the need to use disaster-related funds for health-related disaster research. Funders, Collman said, including FEMA and Congress, need to be educated about why disaster response research is needed and is useful. Funding is needed not only for the study of the clinical and technological aspects of response, but also for the study of organizational management (e.g., coordination, communication, situational assessment, and data sharing). In addition, disasters provide a very specific and unique opportunity to study dose and response in the environmental health field. Funding is needed pre-event to develop infrastructure and instruments and to be ready to arrive at the site as soon as possible and characterize the exposures by whatever means are appropriate (questionnaires, bio-specimens, air monitoring, water monitoring), as the data dissipate exponentially as time passes.

Disaster Risk Reduction and Sustained Investment

Another suggestion was that the nation think programmatically about how to reduce disaster risk. Wenger concurred and noted that the United Nations Office for Disaster Risk Reduction is placing a greater emphasis on disaster mitigation and is developing a post-2015 framework for disaster risk reduction.[8] Several participants also discussed the issue of trust in research and suggested the funding is needed to establish relationships and trust before a disaster through investing in, for example, health infra-structure in a community.

[8]See http://www.unisdr.org/we/coordinate/hfa (accessed November 10, 2014).

BOX 7-1
Rapid and Sustained Funding Mechanisms for Research in Disasters[a]

Challenges and Issues

- Time required to disburse money to applicants, size of awards, and time frame to complete research
- Awareness of sources of funding
- Coordination and implementation needs, financial support, and attention
- Funding needs before disaster: increase infrastructure, baseline data/characterization
- Statutory issues; different disaster funds or sources of funds

Opportunities for Improvement

- Other agencies replicate most successful funding models
- Holistic approaches to rapid response research
- Make sure health is front and center
- Possibilities to fund experts before the disaster and have deployable teams

Critical Partnerships and Collaborations

- Partnering with foundations that are interested in the needs of the communities in order to fill gaps that are necessary to make research impactful
- Community concerns: sustainability, strengthen health systems, and give back to the community

[a]The challenges, opportunities, and partnerships listed were identified by one or more individual participants in this breakout panel discussion. This summary was prepared by the panel facilitator and presented in the subsequent plenary session. This list is not meant to reflect a consensus among workshop participants.

SOURCE: Plenary session summary of breakout panel discussion as reported by panel facilitator Gwen Collman.

There is a need for balance between making the most of the research opportunities that exist only because an incident happens and making overall improvements to the health system. If this is out of balance, the community believes researchers come only when there is a disaster to take information away. Successful research must be couched within the need for health systems strengthening to prevent future events; otherwise, communities have little incentive to support researchers. Investing in systems and infrastructure also means that when disaster strikes, there is already some enhanced capacity of the region to respond and some baseline data (social science, medical, biological).

Various participants discussed the ability of the agencies who already support disaster research to continue to do so given budgetary constraints, and how to engage other funders and replicate other successful funding models. They suggested that a more holistic approach to funding—combining resources to provide funding across a number of areas—could help to reduce duplication and siloed efforts. Partnering with foundations that are interested in local concerns and needs can help to fill critical funding gaps as well as help to make the research experience more palatable and more useful to the community.

8

Improving the Role of Extramural Research Networks

David Abramson of Columbia University's National Center for Disaster Preparedness at the Earth Institute facilitated a discussion on models of extramural research networks that could be used to advance disaster science. Participants discussed the essential role for the academic and clinical research community and other partners in collecting data, data sharing, communications, and other priorities to enable timely research; multiple institutions working together as one entity; and the characteristics of an ongoing, sustained research network.

CONVERGENCE OF MULTIPLE TYPES OF DISASTER RESEARCH

Lori Peek, codirector of the Center for Disaster and Risk Analysis at Colorado State University, stated that social science disaster research likely emerged in the 1920s. The first known empirical study was a doctoral dissertation by Columbia University student Samuel Henry Prince, on the 1917 explosion of a ship in Halifax, Nova Scotia, Canada. His dissertation evaluated the behavioral response to the disaster that claimed many lives and resulted in great environmental destruction. The field was then dormant for about two decades, until World War II and the start of the Cold War sparked an increased interest in human behavior in the face of disaster. From 1949 to 1954, university-based field research teams, led primarily by sociologists, were funded by the military to study a variety of behavioral questions such as: Would people panic in the face of disaster?; Would citizens become so demoralized that they would become incapacitated and unable or unwilling to act?; Would there be civil unrest?; Would there be a need for increased social control? The field teams observed that the answers to all of these questions were generally no, and they wrote extensively about how communities came together and how they shared information to build on preexisting community networks. These early field teams then moved on to study acute onset disasters. The military lost interest in funding these academic research centers, Peek said, but the National Academy of Sciences (NAS) recognized the importance of the work and supported these field research teams through the work of the NAS Committee on Disaster Studies from 1951 through 1962. In 1963, sociologists and disaster researchers, E. L. Quarantelli and Russell Dynes founded the Disaster Research Center, which, Peek noted, recently celebrated its 50th anniversary with a workshop on the state of disaster research and challenges for the future.[1]

Development of Disaster Research Fields

Peek reported on some of the substantive consequences of the development of disaster research that were discussed at the May 2014 Disaster Research Center workshop. Overall, the field has been heavily focused on rapid onset disasters (and correspondingly there has been less focus on slower onset, more chronic types of disasters that also affect many people). The research has been predominantly U.S. focused (although the past decade has shown wider scope). In general, disaster research has used classical social science research methods to understand collective responses to disaster. The social science disaster research community has been focused on applied concerns and policy outcomes, Peek said. The theoretical base that is available is predominately grounded in sociology, with a focus on collective behavior and organizational response, and on demographic disparities and social vulnerability.

Peek noted that there has been tremendous growth in the field of social science disaster research over the past five or six decades. The field now incorporates natural hazards research; engineering, atmospheric science, computer science, and other technical fields; public health research; and science, technology, and society research. Having attended several recent meetings on disaster research, Peek observed that the same conversations and the same calls for action are occurring in each of these domains, in particular, the need for websites to compile information datasets, ready-made research protocols, and lists of experts (rosters) so that teams can be more rapidly assembled after a disaster (similar needs experts were asking at this current workshop). The question is how all of these domains can

[1]See http://www.udel.edu/DRC (accessed December 18, 2014).

mobilize together in such a way as to influence national, state, and local policy to reduce disaster losses.

As an example of mobilizing diverse partners, Peek described the Social Science Research Council Task Force on Hurricane Katrina and Rebuilding the Gulf Coast. The thinking of the task force from the beginning was that Hurricane Katrina was too big of an event to conduct the usual one-off case studies and short-term studies that provide only a snapshot of a particular element of a tremendous event, she said. Hurricane Katrina was such a multidimensional event that there was no one person and no one discipline alone that could truly understand it. Similarly, disaster research could benefit from multiple disciplines working together, combining both clinical and social sciences.

> If we could actually work together as teams and try to understand the disaster in a much more complex way, rather than creating just a tile, we could have a mosaic.
>
> —*Lori Peek*

Following a series of meetings along the Gulf Coast with researchers, workers on the ground, and community members, the task force developed a program of 10 distinct studies spanning an array of topics from risk communication, to environmental impacts, to displaced populations. Peek explained that the studies were independent but done in conversation with one another. The Social Science Research Council provided support for a website where researchers posted profiles of their work so others could find who was doing what research on Hurricane Katrina by a keyword search. The council also provided briefings or short bulletins to inform the practice communities about the research findings in a timely manner. The long-term vision is to produce the Katrina Bookshelf, including books on each of the independently funded projects together in an edited collection. Peek noted that the first book on population displacement after Hurricane Katrina has been released, three more are in press (children in Katrina, cultural trauma, environmental and community impacts), and the remaining books are in development.[2]

---

[2]See http://utpress.utexas.edu/index.php/books/series/series/The-Katrina-Bookshelf (accessed December 18, 2014).

ADVANCING SCIENCE DURING CRISIS

Gary Machlis, coleader of the Strategic Sciences Group (SSG) at the U.S. Department of the Interior (DOI), discussed characteristics of, and recommendations for, advancing science during crisis (i.e., while it is happening, not in preparation for or in response to). As background, he explained that the SSG was formed by secretarial order following an experimental deployment during the Deepwater Horizon disaster. The mission of the SSG is limited to conducting interdisciplinary, science-based assessments and scenario building during a major environmental crisis and delivering the results and potential interventions to decision makers. The SSG uses interdisciplinary teams of both federal and nonfederal personnel. Machlis explained that the SSG drew some of its organizational principles from the research and development division of the World War II intelligence agency, the Office of Strategic Services. Those principles include focus on the mission, not the process; build operational teams based on expertise, not representation, and on skill, not rank; and have direct access to leaders and decision makers. Machlis also noted the value of having personnel with both physical and mental strength when working in disaster research.

Characteristics in Crisis to Include

Based on the work of the SSG, Machlis outlined six distinctive characteristics of science during crisis that could be included in a research framework focused on health.

- **Coupled human and natural systems.** Science in crisis is to inform response, and responses with significant consequences require coupled human and natural systems approaches. A purely biophysical or purely sociocultural approach is ineffective. The ability to deliver actionable recommendations is limited by science in silos because real-world decisions transcend human and natural systems.
- **Collaboration and interdisciplinary teams.** A coupled human and natural systems approach relies on interdisciplinary teams. However, a disaster often brings together people who do not know each other or who do not have a long history of working together. The critical challenge is to create, within hours, a working interdisciplinary team of the best expertise available. Team

members must work using the same vocabulary; suspend their own territorial claims, disciplinary turf, and paradigms of thought; and work for the common good.

- **Uncertainties and limitations.** It is not sufficient to deliver findings to decision makers unless they are accompanied by a clear presentation of the uncertainties and limitations of the findings, Machlis said. The SSG uses a scientific scale of uncertainty based on that of the Intergovernmental Panel on Climate Change.
- **Cascading consequences and assessing impacts.** Crises often have an immediate need for tactical science (e.g., how to cap a leaking oil well), but it is important to remember that decisions regarding the emergency response will influence long-term restoration as well. There is a need to understand the cascade of consequences of each decision, each of which has its own uncertainty.
- **Sense of place.** While crises have commonalities, every crisis is distinct from the next, and all disasters are local. Having a sense of place is vital to success, Machlis stressed. It is not enough, for example, to have demographic data on the populations or neighborhoods that might be affected. What is required is an understanding of cultural history and a visceral sense of place.
- **Communicating science during crisis.** Communication during crisis requires extraordinary clarity and concise explanation of the findings, uncertainties, and implications. This is much more important than the literature review, background, or methods. Compelling visualization is also essential to convey the message (e.g., maps, graphs, figures, charts). In addition, when communicating with leadership, researchers must speak the truth and be transparent, without ambushing them through public attention seeking.

Machlis concluded by offering four recommendations for advancing science in crisis:

1. Identify best practices of science during crisis.
2. Advance systematic rostering by learning from others who use it (e.g., the U.S. Forest Service for fighting wildfires).
3. Seek legislative relief from the Federal Advisory Committee Act (FACA) provisions that prohibit or impede federal/non-federal scientific collaboration in a disaster. A presidential disaster

declaration should trigger a FACA exemption for certain forms of scientific work.

4. Prepare leadership before a crisis to be ready to integrate science into decision making during a crisis.

PHARMACEUTICAL RESEARCH DURING A DISASTER

Paul Seligman, executive director for Global Regulatory Policy at Amgen, offered a pharmaceutical company perspective on disaster research. A pharmaceutical company that sponsors a product for U.S. regulatory approval first conducts or sponsors clinical studies of the product and then uses that data (and possibly data from others) to assemble a dossier and submit an application for marketing approval to FDA. Sponsors develop the product labeling and conduct additional postapproval studies. With regard to disaster preparedness, sponsors provide and maintain products for the Strategic National Stockpile (SNS), both prespecified quantities purchased by the SNS as well as product for surge capacity and stock rotation to maintain maximum shelf life. He reminded participants that under the Animal Rule, FDA can approve a drug or biologic product based on substantial evidence of efficacy from studies in animals when efficacy studies in humans are not ethical or feasible.[3]

Seligman noted that companies have a lot of information about their products that may not be in the public domain, for example, analytics particular to measuring levels of the product; additional data on product parameters (e.g., pharmacokinetics, pharmacodynamics, genetic testing/susceptibility, biomarkers); or data from clinical trials regarding other potential indications, specific treated populations, or other comparators, including historical controls. This means, Seligman suggested that pharmaceutical sponsors may have baseline information of interest to disaster researchers, albeit in the context of the development of their product for an indication that is used in medicine generally.

The immediate response to any event will be managed by public health, the medical field, law enforcement, and the disaster and response infrastructure, Seligman concluded. While the sponsor's role is generally to ensure supply of medicine, there are a variety of opportunities for collaboration with pharmaceutical product sponsors before, during, and after a disaster. A sponsor's role extends, for example, to the development of the postevent study protocols, contribution of unique analytic

[3]21 CFR 314.600 (drugs) and 21 CFR 601.90 (biologics).

capabilities, involvement in the conduct and analysis of studies, and patient communications, but they may not realize this until engaged and asked for assistance.

RESPONSE TO ENVIRONMENTAL HEALTH IMPACTS OF DISASTERS

Sharon Croisant, director of the Community Outreach and Education Core at the University of Texas Medical Branch (UTMB) Center in Environmental Toxicology, shared several examples of UTMB's evolving involvement in research efforts in the field in direct response to disasters. The research efforts of the Community Outreach and Education Core after Hurricanes Isaac, Katrina, and Rita started simply, she said, by contacting Red Cross and community shelters to compile lists of supplies that people needed (e.g., water, mosquito repellant, adhesive bandages, antibiotics) and then collecting and delivering those supplies. This grew into informal needs assessments in the communities, which turned into a year-long project to assess community resiliency and preparedness. Similar needs assessments and relief and response efforts were done in Galveston after Hurricane Ike. In addition, there was a community-based participatory research project focused on assessing toxins in the posthurricane sediment sludge. Croisant noted that when the waters receded, sludge was left behind in three-quarters of the residential and commercial buildings on Galveston Island. Much of the floodwaters came from the bay, which she said is contaminated with pollutants from Superfund sites, an old creosote plant, a sewage plant, a sulfur repository, and the port. The findings (toxins including arsenic, cadmium, chromium, and others) were important not only for the residents, but also for those involved in the cleanup (tens of thousands of people on the island mucking out homes and doing repairs, including 5,000 college students who came to Galveston over a period of 2 years to help clean up). Safety training sessions were held for the volunteers, and an educational series on mold and lead paint was also developed. Croisant added that materials were translated into Spanish, as many of the workers and families did not speak English.

Creating a Consortium

As a result of its work in the aftermath of the hurricanes, UTMB had established relationships with the Gulf Coast communities of Texas.

Croisant said that after the Deepwater Horizon explosion and oil spill, those communities began calling and expressing concern about the conflicting information they were hearing from the White House, the media, the National Oceanic Atmospheric Administration, and others. UTMB conducted scoping visits to better understand their fears. Efforts were made to find and report back with answers, and an NIEHS U19 consortium project was established to study the health risks related to the spill. The consortium included academic institutions as well as community groups from the impacted areas (e.g., Vietnamese Fisherfolk, United Houma Nation, Alabama Fisheries Cooperative, and Bayou Interfaith Shared Community Organizing). The mission of the consortium was to explore the health impacts and the community resiliency related to the Deepwater Horizon disaster by fostering collaborative interactions among multi-disciplinary, multi-institutional, basic, and clinical investigators, supported by active involvement of community partners. Because the project involved seafood sampling, those partners included, for example, shrimpers, commercial fishermen, and people running the seafood processing market. Croisant noted that around 350 fishermen were trained to collect samples. A total of 24 community meetings revealed that people were most concerned about the safety of the seafood. They needed to know definitively if it was contaminated and could not be sold or eaten, or if it was safe and how to get that message out to everyone. The consortium is studying the presence and toxicity of petrogenic polycyclic aromatic hydrocarbons, evaluating exposures and longitudinal outcomes, and disseminating findings to the community stakeholders.

Barriers Encountered

Croisant highlighted several challenges to getting out into the field in a timely manner. Funding must be repurposed or solicited and may involve multiple industry and agency stakeholders. Bureaucracy is an impediment, she said; for example, getting a new vendor approved when a suitable vendor is not already in the system takes too much time. The lack of a communications infrastructure means that information is fragmented and intermittent. Coordination among local, state, and federal agencies sometimes lacks infrastructure and thus impedes communication and integration of efforts. Communities are rarely prepared for disasters, and poor communities are the least resilient, Croisant added.

Another concern is that emergency responders generally lack training on possible environmental exposures (e.g., toxins in the sediment sludge after Hurricane Ike). In addition, emissions or spills resulting from flooding or accidents are frequently not identified until much too late to protect public health. Croisant also noted that there can be tension between and among community members and groups, industry, science, and government that can intensify in emergency situations. Technology can be a barrier, particularly when it is not available as a result of the disaster. For example, cell phone service is often interrupted, and fewer and fewer people have landlines. Internet service can also be disrupted, limiting access to emergency information generally found online (e.g., Material Safety Data Sheets) or limiting the ability of people to sign up for services and assistance online.

Moving forward, UTMB has been working on developing a partnership with the Galveston County network of regional Emergency Management representatives, leveraging emergency management training and integrating UTMB Center in Environmental Toxicology resources.

CHALLENGES AND OPPORTUNITIES

In summarizing the panel discussions, Abramson said that a framework for an extramural research community collaborative could include multidisciplinary strategic science teams, consortia, suppliers, and intra- and interdisciplinary research networks (see Box 8-1). It is important to recognize that many networks already exist, Croisant said, and she recommended working to integrate those. There is also already a cadre of scientific experts at NIEHS core centers, Clinical and Translational Science Award institutes, and other centers. The question is how to identify those that would be appropriate and willing to participate in a disaster response research network. As part of networking for preparedness, Machlis said, researchers need to learn about the scales larger and smaller than the one at which they work. For example, an ecologist might work with a watershed area, or an ecosystem, or a region, or large landscape, or a sociologist might work at the level of a family, or neighborhood, or larger community.

When a crisis happens, it is valuable to know how we are connected to those working at the scale above and below. A key challenge is identifying who can bring all of these entities together and coordinate efforts. It was discussed that coordinating bodies could be the mission agencies (e.g., CDC or DOI), funders (e.g., NIH, NSF, foundations), or regulators (e.g., FDA).

BOX 8-1
Improving Extramural Research Collaboration[a]

Challenges and Issues

- Research can operate as:
  - Teams (multidisciplinary strategic science teams)
  - Consortia (addressing/engaging community partners)
  - Suppliers (e.g., medical countermeasures; public–private partners)
  - Broad networks (both intra- and interdisciplinary)
- Who can organize and coordinate these collaboratives?

Opportunities for Improvement

- Recommendations for regulatory relief (FACA)
- Pilot-test the system

Critical Partnerships and Collaborations

- Mission agencies (CDC, DOI)
- Funders (NIH, NSF, foundations)
- Regulators (FDA)
- Can we "crowdsource" solutions to the most significant problems (through the Internet)?

[a]The challenges, opportunities, and partnerships listed were identified by one or more individual participants in this breakout panel discussion. This summary was prepared by the panel facilitator and presented in the subsequent plenary session. This list is not meant to reflect a consensus among workshop participants.

SOURCE: Plenary session summary of breakout panel discussion as reported by panel facilitator David Abramson.

Seligman raised a concern that it is not clear what agency or group a pharmaceutical company could engage to ensure that adequate information on benefit and safety is going to be collected when the company's product is used in a disaster response. Industry is developing medical countermeasures with an FDA requirement to have protocols in place so that when those products are used, data are captured regarding effectiveness and safety of the product. Where in the public health community or in the academic community would a pharmaceutical company turn to ensure that capturing that kind of information is included in protocols and instruments that are being developed? It was suggested by some that there be a more focused discussion, perhaps a follow-up workshop, on the issue of collecting postmarket product data in a crisis response.

Irwin Redlener, director of the National Center for Disaster Preparedness at Columbia University, said there is no public health infrastructure in the United States that has an authoritative overview of what the country's priorities are relative to nearly every aspect of preparedness, including how to ensure the collection of data on the use of pharmaceutical products in a crisis. There is no infrastructure that allows the government to answer a broad, important public health question simply, clearly, definitively, and quickly. He suggested that one reason we keep repeating the same mistakes and not learning lessons is a lack of a fundamental structural organization for dealing with disasters.

Moving forward, a participant called for regulatory relief from FACA and other provisions that might impede scientific collaboration in a disaster. Abramson also called for pilot-testing the system before the disaster occurs, setting up small collaboratives at multiple levels and working on fictional scenarios and directed tabletop exercises to become well practiced at rapidly bringing partners together across disciplinary spans. It was also suggested that it might be possible to crowdsource solutions, engaging not only the science community but the greater public.

9

Coordinating Logistics to Execute Rapid Research in Disaster Response

This section focuses on the logistics of rapid research in a disaster, with discussions facilitated by Howard Zucker, acting commissioner of health for the state of New York. Participants discussed triggers for go/no-go scenarios, just-in-time training for research responders, integration of disaster research response into the ICS, and corresponding logistical needs when working in disaster settings.

INTEGRATING DISASTER RESEARCH INTO THE INCIDENT COMMAND STRUCTURE

From a state and local agency perspective, disaster research should inform or enhance emergency response or recovery activities, said Shelley DuTeaux, the assistant deputy director for public health and emergency preparedness for the California Department of Public Health. All disasters are local, she said, whether the locality is a neighborhood, a city or county, or multiple cities or counties. In a disaster, if localities lack or have exhausted their resources and capabilities, they will request assistance from a county or regional level. If they cannot assist, the request elevates to the state level (or state-to-state mutual aid through agreements such as an Emergency Management Assistance Compact) and then to the federal level.

Each state should have an ICS, which is a tool for coordinating resources and communication during an emergency. The ICS is integrated throughout the emergency management structure. All response and recovery activities (federal, state, mutual aid) are done in support of the local activities, and activities should integrate into the emergency management structure that is already in place. In this regard, anyone who brings research resources to the field needs to know and integrate into the emergency management structure, DuTeaux said. She recommended that researchers planning to go in the field get basic training on the ICS so they know where they fit into the emergency operations structure and do not hinder the response.[1] In particular, in the ICS there is an incident safety officer who is responsible for the safety of everyone in the field, and researchers should make their presence in the field known to the safety officer.

All states have different thresholds and capacity at which they may request federal assistance. Requests may be made in the case of a presidential declaration of emergency (a Stafford Act declaration authorizing the delivery of federal technical, financial, logistical, and other assistance during a declared disaster or emergency). Federal assistance, coordinated by FEMA, is provided if the governor certifies that the event exceeds the combined response capabilities of the state and local governments. DuTeaux pointed out that the presidential emergency declaration specifies the type of assistance authorized, and therefore, for assistance for disaster research to be authorized, it must be in the emergency declaration.

If there is no presidential declaration, access to federal assistance can still be given directly through the appropriate agency if that agency has the authority to act and to expend its own resources. The U.S. Environmental Protection Agency (EPA), for example, can act on its own authority with its own money to help states in the absence of a presidential declaration. DuTeaux noted that in the midst of an emergency, the state might not know what federal resources are available to it. It would help, she suggested, if federal partners would "lean forward" and suggest the kind of help they can provide.

In closing, DuTeaux noted that data collected during disaster response research could potentially be used in an enforcement action. Data should be secured, and researchers should follow up with local response and recovery authorities on next steps and leave their contact information with the community and local public health authority.

---

[1]Free training courses through FEMA can be found at http://training.fema.gov/emiweb/is/icsresource/index.htm (accessed February 4, 2015).

RAPID RESEARCH: THE U.S. CRITICAL ILLNESS AND INJURY TRIALS GROUP

The U.S. Critical Illness and Injury Trials Group (USCIITG) entered disaster and preparedness research because of its interest in rapid identification of and intervention in life- threatening situations, said Charles Cairns, associate director of USCIITG. This application is similar to public health practice and disaster epidemiology, discussed in Chapter 7. For example, the group implemented a heart attack system that reduced mortality across the state of North Carolina by getting everyone treated within 90 minutes, independent of where they were at the time of their heart attack or their hospital system affiliation. USCIITG is a "network of networks," including established research networks and professional organizations and more than 200 investigators across 68 intensive care units in U.S. hospitals. USCIITG has four main programs focused on identifying and enrolling patients within minutes of their intersection with the health care system: Prevention of Organ Failure; Critical Illness Outcomes Study; Early Intensive Care Unit (ICU) Rehabilitation; and Program for Emergency Preparedness (PREP).

The aim of PREP is to "significantly enhance the national capability to rapidly glean crucial information regarding the clinical course of acute illness and injury and guide clinical resource requirements during emergent events." The goal is to not only collect these data, but to analyze them quickly and disseminate the results, ideally within 24 hours. Most of the datasets are geared to be done in a minute or two, Cairns said, and would be considered very minimal from the point of view of a specialty researcher; however, the way their approach is done is "better than perfect." Cairns listed several of the key clinical outcomes and operational questions to be addressed by the data:

- What was the nature of the clinical insult and the resulting phenotype?
- As a clinical responder, what, if anything, did you have to do differently?
- Did clinical diagnostics, countermeasures, and therapies work as expected?
- What was the operational impact on the patient and care setting?
- Was there anything essential needed that you did not get?
- What is the best/worst case that could happen next time?

The first step to working with a rapid response clinical research network in a public health emergency is to define a key dataset. An all-hazard minimum dataset was defined as applicable to all phases of care (prehospital, emergency department, intensive care unit, discharge/follow-up, rehabilitation). The NIH Research Electronic Data Capture system was used so that the data could be collected using a smart device and would also be accessible to an analytic system. Specialized datasets were then developed, addressing specific hazards (infectious diseases, radiation injury, traumatic injury).

> We see emergencies every day on a large scale. If we can leverage that experience, knowledge, and infrastructure, we should be able to conduct sound research, we should be able to analyze it quickly, and of course, through professional organizations and clinical care structures, disseminate the results rapidly.
>
> —*Charles Cairns*

A clinical feasibility pilot study was then done to test the concepts and "field usability" of the core dataset in an everyday setting (burn injuries). The pilot also assessed the logistics of human subjects research in a public health emergency, especially IRB approval. Cairns reported that within 24 hours, 195 patients were enrolled across 12 sites, data were collected and reported to the coordination center, and analysis was disseminated, showing that it is possible to perform and share rapid assessments.

A key challenge highlighted by the pilot study was the IRB process, specifically, what was defined as research for the purposes of the IRB review, the time frames for review, and the variance in responses. These issues need to be addressed if we are to conduct clinically meaningful interventional research on time-sensitive, life-threatening illness and injury, Cairns said. Moving forward, he recommended reliance agreements in conjunction with an operational PHERRB (discussed at greater length earlier in this summary). Other considerations moving forward include the need for standardized data elements and reporting platforms for public health emergencies and coordinated international networks.

In conclusion, Cairns said that emergencies happen every day on a large scale. If we can leverage that experience, knowledge, and infrastructure, we should be able to conduct sound research, analyze it quickly, and disseminate the results rapidly through professional organizations and clinical care structures.

FEDERAL PERSPECTIVE ON LOGISTICS FOR RAPID DISASTER RESEARCH RESPONSE

The NIEHS Worker Education and Training Program is authorized under the Superfund Amendments and Reauthorization Act of 1986 to provide competitive training grants in hazardous waste removal and containment, and emergency responses involving toxic substances. The WETP Emergency Support Activation Plan is built on the protocols of the Worker Safety and Health Annex of the National Response Framework (NRF). Hughes of NIEHS noted that of the 15 Emergency Support Functions (ESFs) of the NRF, much of the NIEHS work over the years has been under ESF 8, Public Health and Medical Services (for which HHS is the lead) and ESF 10, Oil and Hazardous Materials Response (for which EPA is the lead). He suggested that disaster research could be built into the ESF structure, for example, public health research as part of ESF 8.

When a disaster happens, decisions about exposure and protection of first responders, workers, or communities often happen in a silo because the site-safety officer is disconnected to what might be happening in the field. Decisions are made based on the best data and information available at the moment. The earlier we can bring in better information, the better we can ensure that people do not engage in risky activities, Hughes said. The challenge is how to get information to people in the field when research information about hazards becomes available.

One approach to protecting workers is through site-specific training materials (see Figure 9-1). The NIEHS disaster response to the WTC collapses on 9/11 included, for example, on-site training for more than 7,000 response workers.

Deepwater Horizon oil spill response was another situation where instantaneous decisions about protection and risk had to be made, Hughes said. Just-in-time field training was provided for 150,000 people through short courses in English, Spanish, and Vietnamese. Training materials were developed by WETP together with BP, NIOSH, and the Occupational Safety and Health Administration (OSHA), and more than 35,000 training books were distributed.[2]

In response to Hurricane Sandy, WETP coordinated with OSHA and other agencies to provide site hazard assessments and develop site-

[2]Available at https://www.osha.gov/Publications/Oil_Spill_Booklet_05.11_v4.pdf (accessed December 18, 2014).

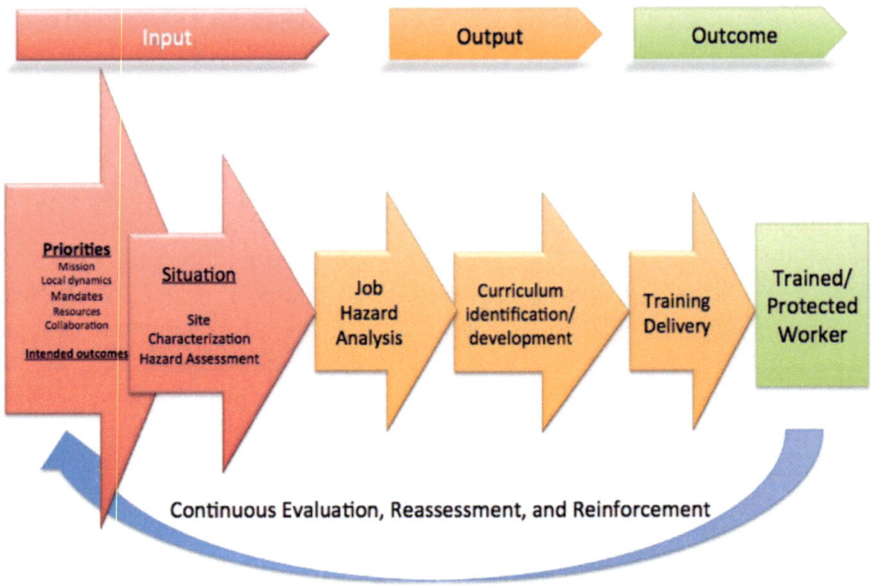

FIGURE 9-1 Site-specific training development.
SOURCE: Hughes presentation, June 13, 2014.

provided in-classroom, site-specific health and safety training for more than 3,000 cleanup workers, and hundreds of hours of technical assistance, training, and briefings were provided on-site.

In closing, Hughes concurred with the need to determine how research fits into the emergency response structure and the importance of connections to the ICS. Research should be ready to go, with pretrained responders, he said, and the acute response should help provide a foundation for further research (e.g., sample collection for later use, surveillance activities).

MAKING RESEARCH USEFUL TO THE RESPONSE

A critical gap in disaster research is during the disaster and immediately after impact, said Joseph Barbera, codirector of the Institute for Crisis, Disaster and Risk Management at George Washington University. Much of current research focuses on the predisaster and later postdisaster time frames, and there is a fair amount of disinformation around medical problems that occur within the first hours after an event. The challenge is how to conduct good research in the immediate postimpact period when everything is chaotic, or at least recognize the limitations to close the gap as much as possible.

Collecting Perishable Data

Barbera emphasized the issue of perishable data. In a disaster, the scale, scope, and chaos can obscure the detail. Following an earthquake in the Philippines in 1990, for example, Baguio City in Luzon Province was completely isolated by landslides caused by the earthquakes. The only way in was by military aircraft. In addition to full-scale search and rescue, Barbera was trying to gather data from the three area hospitals for the Office of Foreign Disaster Assistance on which to base donation decisions. Barbera described the challenges of getting accurate information about how many patients the three local hospitals took care of in the first 24 hours after the earthquake. One hospital simply had no idea, as they cared for so many they were not even keeping track.

With perishable data there is also the issue of honest and unvarnished reporting versus processed and rationalized reporting, Barbera said. The raw story is the first time it is told, versus the polished version it becomes after many retellings. This is human behavior, often unintentional, and happens to everyone as our brains start to remember things differently, or the uncertainty starts to become less uncertain. This is why it is especially important to try to capture data rapidly in a sudden onset incident. Another phenomenon that is important to recognize when trying to capture data from a sudden onset incident is that the information reported can also evolve over time depending on why it is being provided. The story may lean one way early on when people or organizations are seeking assistance, and another way later when they are seeking to reduce potential liability (e.g., for performance during the disaster).

Barbera emphasized that part of data collection is also capturing the emergency context so that there can be accurate data interpretation. For example, Barbera shared how a man survived for 15 days buried in rubble following an earthquake in the Philippines in 1990 as a result of how the building collapsed and because rainwater was available. However, the situation was different after the earthquake in Haiti and searches were called off earlier as no further survivors were expected.

Sensitivities and Competencies

Sending researchers into disasters raises a variety of issues. The first concern highlighted by Barbera, and other speakers throughout this report, is the perception of research during a disaster. A situation is classified as a disaster because it exceeds resources, and research resources are often viewed as replacing response resources. Thus it is important to consider the relevancy of the research. Another issue is sensitivity, as the people impacted can feel that U.S. researchers come to their country and do research on their misfortunes so that the information can be used to help people in the researchers' own country. There can also be similar sensitivities in local responses. Competency is another issue, and Barbera related it to the points made by DuTeaux about integrating research with the ICS. Researchers can be seen as interfering with or skewing the response, or potentially skewing later assessment of the response decisions and actions. Barbera told participants to think about how they would feel if firefighters had to respond to an incident in their research lab where all of their equipment and work is, and then to think of how firefighters might feel about researchers coming into an incident while they were working. Researchers might not be as physically destructive, he said, but could be every bit as functionally destructive.

One potential solution to these challenges, Barbera suggested, is to train responders to capture research data, although he acknowledged there are positives and negatives to that approach. Another approach, as noted by others, is for researchers to gain an operational level of proficiency with and participate in the ICS. One place for researchers to consider engaging is in the planning section of the ICS, in particular, the situation unit and the technical specialist unit. The planning section supports, promotes, and executes the development of the incident action plan for the next operational period. The situation unit is charged with capturing the data, particularly from the operation section, and putting that into a format that can inform decisions during the incident and action planning process. The data that might need to be collected to understand the situation at the action planning level are also data that could be very useful in research. Barbera added that collecting good data for the purposes of improvement of response might not need IRB approval and that data could be used later for research. Barbera noted that many of the ICS forms used for incident action planning contain data that could be used for research.

To study sudden onset events, researchers need to be able to deploy rapidly and have reliable transport to the incident. They need to know how to check in with and integrate into the ICS even if they are "just doing research," as this helps to build a trust relationship. Researchers also need to have an operational level of proficiency regarding safety and protective equipment, as well as other knowledge and skills relevant to operating in the disaster area (emphasizing DuTeaux's earlier point around training in the ICS principles). It is also important that researchers understand the need to be self-sustaining (e.g., with regard to food, water, lodging/billeting). Barbera expressed concerns about "disaster tourism," or people masquerading as researchers or clinicians. Researchers do not necessarily need to be at the scene, Barbera noted. Access to data could be facilitated through the emergency operation centers, for example, which directly support the incident management team. Researchers might also have services to offer the operations centers in terms of analyzing data in real time.

Overall, researchers should strive to be of use to the response, helping to collect data and rapidly disseminate raw aggregate information for use by appropriate responders. Be available to provide competent (i.e., situational) technical advice while conducting the research mission, and contribute to situation reports for incident action planning. Finally, Barbera said, consider this to be applied research. The disaster response becomes the research proof of concept for years of very intensive planning, peer review, and research. If we can understand these disaster contexts, we can develop useful strategies and tools and test the proofs of concept when they are needed (recognizing that there should be alternate plans that can be immediately implemented if the proof is not obtained).

CHALLENGES AND OPPORTUNITIES

A point reiterated throughout the discussion was the need to integrate research into the emergency response structure; Cairns reported in summarizing the session (see Box 9-1). There were discussions of public health integrating with state agencies and local responses, understanding where research fits into the ICS, and understanding that there are both operational and safety components that need to be addressed.

Another key issue was the need to identify the research priorities and key questions, and then develop data collection systems and train researchers, responders, and other partners to rapidly collect data to answer those questions. For example, Cairns said, do we want to understand the

BOX 9-1
Coordinating Logistics to Execute Rapid Research in a Response[a]

Challenges and Issues

- Integration with response structures and systems (ICS)
- Identify research questions and outcomes
- Capture immediate information (training, rapid data collection and systems)

Opportunities for Improvement

- Integrate research into elements of the Emergency Support Functions (ESFs)
- Centralized support for human subjects research (reliance agreements, PHERRB)
- Incorporate research into response training
- Develop a national research response framework

Critical Partnerships and Collaborations

- Response elements (local, state, federal)
- Trainers across multiple response dimension
- Federal research institutions (NIH, CDC, NSF, nonhealth)

[a]The challenges, opportunities, and partnerships listed were identified by one or more individual participants in this breakout panel discussion. This summary was prepared by the panel facilitator and presented in the subsequent plenary session. This list is not meant to reflect a consensus among workshop participants.

SOURCE: Plenary session summary of breakout panel discussion as reported by panel presenter Charles Cairns on behalf of facilitator Howard Zucker.

event; understand the systems of care and management; develop new interventions? The value of applied research is that it can help to answer immediate questions relevant to the response and provide decision makers with key information for allocating resources and meeting people's needs, but it is also foundational data for later research and can inform policies and procedures going forward. Some participants highlighted the immediate post impact period as one of the information gaps in disasters and stressed the need to collect "perishable" data rapidly and to collect contextual information associated with the data as well.

Cairns suggested that disaster research could be built into the ESF structure, particularly the public health–focused ESFs. A participant noted that the science required for response preparedness and recovery crosscuts all of the ESFs. The tendency is to focus on the health piece, but to be successful there needs to be a national research framework that includes everyone, local through federal, and public and private partners.

Part of the logistical network for disaster research would be centralized support for human subjects research, and similar to the IRB conversation, a few participants discussed the PHERRB and reliance agreements. The need for a national research response framework was also discussed, potentially integrating the elements of human subjects protection, minimum datasets, standardized terminology and processes, research training, the ICS, and public health emergency structures at the local, state, and national levels.

10

Actions to Build the Future of Disaster Research

In this final chapter, experts offer remarks about the issues and opportunities raised throughout the summary, including commenting on some of the challenges highlighted at the end of each chapter. They considered strategies for improved inclusion and integration of all stakeholders to support the timely identification of health research priorities, collection of data to understand health impacts, efficacy of responses, and risk factors to strengthen resiliency and future preparedness.

DEFINING THE KEY QUESTIONS AND THE CORE DATASET

Reflecting on the workshop, Paul Biddinger, medical director for emergency preparedness at Massachusetts General Hospital and Partners Healthcare, suggested that there is a need to be bold but restrained. Often, he said, it is hard to have concrete items to follow up on after such a broad set of ideas and questions has been put forth in the workshop discussions. As discussed throughout the workshop, it is incumbent on the research community to come up with the key questions that need to be answered and an agreed-to core set of data elements needed to answer those questions. These elements must be captured in an event by everyone, and he suggested that the core set of data elements could be built into the ICS forms, CMS reporting requirements, Joint Commission accreditation requirements, and the like. The worse the chaos gets, the more you lose your data, he said. As noted by others, trying to recreate the data after the event is not nearly the same thing.

Marcia McNutt, the editor in chief of *Science*, emphasized the need to keep the end goal in mind when defining the questions, which is using science to ultimately reduce disaster risk and improve disaster mitigation. It is important to understand what happened during the event, why it led to human impact, and how to interrupt the cascade of consequences that led to negative impacts on humans. The most important disaster is often the one no one hears about because it was prevented. An example, McNutt said, is the 2002 magnitude 7.9 earthquake on the Denali fault that ruptured right beneath the Trans-Alaska pipeline, and not a drop of oil was spilled. She suggested that disaster was averted as a result of decades of work by seismologists to understand the ground motion from earthquakes, which led to the earthquake-proof design of the pipeline (S-curves on sliders to allow for movement). She acknowledged, however, the challenges of funding for research to prevent disasters. The interest in such research is greatest immediately after a disaster, but it can quickly wane, and true, validated answers can take time.

> The most important disaster is the one that never made the headline because you prevented it from happening, because of all the science you did and all the mitigation you did, and so no one ever knew about it.
>
> —*Marcia McNutt*

Sally Phillips, acting principal deputy assistant secretary in the Office of Health Affairs at the U.S. Department of Homeland Security, also reiterated the need for a set of core data elements that should be collected and the need for a central repository for the data. We don't need everybody asking the same questions over and over again, she said.

DATA COLLECTION: BUILDING DAY-TO-DAY SYSTEMS, NETWORKS, AND TRUST

McNutt highlighted the need to institutionalize networks with a diversity of partners and partnerships. One way to achieve this, she suggested, is to integrate networks into day-to-day operations, rather than having them for use in emergencies only. Activities such as gathering routine baseline data in collaboration with partners set up networks that can be tapped in emergencies. Other ways to build networks are through exercising scenarios, risk communication activities, and educational events. Biddinger suggested that a national program modeled on the Medical Reserve Corps program could help to address the manpower shortages in a disaster. A "research reserve corps" would be volunteers who are trained and ready to help collect data during a disaster in a manner that would not detract from the response.

Sally Phillips concurred with comments made during the workshop that anyone can be trained to collect data and do it well, as long as there are quality assurances in place. How can we empower citizen researchers in a disaster to start gathering baseline data (being careful not to burden those who are overwhelmed with the event)? She suggested, for example, that people in shelters who cannot yet return home are often extremely bored and might make good citizen scientists. Engaging the citizenry not only in gathering information, but in taking action on the results, improves the resilience and the responsiveness of the community.

Phillips also reminded participants of the discussions around trust and the need to ensure that the data collection process protects the privacy of the people and the community, especially during a crisis when they are most vulnerable. Trust is central, Irwin Redlener reiterated, and it must not be squandered by asking questions that are not going to be meaningful or by not engaging to use the findings to influence public policy.

Biddinger also raised the issue of health systems research and noted that there are certain elements of research about systems that can only be captured during a disaster. The response in Boston to the Boston Marathon bombings had a lot to do with systems, he said, and there is no question that a lot of what was done should be credited to research. Boston modified its disaster plans years ago after considering the data from responses to mass casualty incidents around the world.

SCIENTISTS AS ADVOCATES

Irwin Redlener of Columbia University raised concerns about the ability of research to influence policy, citing a spate of recent disasters that could have been avoided, lessened, or responded to more effectively if lessons from prior disasters had been heeded or scientific knowledge about the phenomena had been taken into account and changes or plans made.

He recommended that any proposal to any agency that deals with preparedness should have a justification for why the research program will prepare for, prevent, or mitigate disasters and save lives. The ultimate goal is to substantially reduce the risk of people dying in disasters and improve the chances of a rapid, efficient recovery from disasters. Everything has to feed in to that agenda, he said. He called for a strategic national plan that outlines where research fits in a purposeful way.

Redlener listed three barriers to full preparedness: federalism (which prohibits the federal government from requiring particular preparedness actions unless it is a national emergency); bureaucracy and dysfunctional relationships between and among federal, state, and city agencies; and gaps between science and policy and between the private sector and government.

To address the gap between science and policy, Redlener called for a new level of activism by scientists for dealing with the big issues. Preparedness plans made in the absence of key information are insufficient, and scientists must step up and be heard by policy makers, especially with regard to issues of scale. He mentioned as an example the efforts by New York State on pandemic influenza preparedness, and opined that the commitment was insufficient by a factor of 10 based on the actual needs of hospitals. Research needs to extend into what the consequences of the findings may be, or how concerns can be fixed. Somebody has to do it, and right now nobody is, he said.

> I don't think there should be any federal funding for any kind of [disaster] research that doesn't have a goal of saving lives and guiding policy.
>
> —*Irwin Redlener*

Engaging with Policy Makers

Sally Phillips concurred with the need to be politically active, but noted that researchers are often reluctant to engage in the political environment. Policy makers will incorporate research into policy if it is conveyed to them in a way they can understand it, on an ongoing basis, she said. They will not read it in journals. She suggested that sharing information can help to mobilize the political structure to the scientist's favor. For example, funding usually follows disaster events, but it rarely includes research money (supplemental funding following Hurricane Sandy being a recent exception, with some research funding included in the appropriations). She suggested that if the political structure is made aware of the research being conducted during disasters, and the ongoing, long-term data being collected, there could be more research funding targeted in supplemental appropriations related to these disasters. Researchers cannot be shy about sharing data and cannot wait to share with policy makers until

> Policy makers will incorporate your research into their policy, if you bother to tell it to them in a way they can understand it, on an ongoing basis.
>
> —*Sally Phillips*

it is perfect and ready for publication. Biddinger added that it is also important to publicize when research leads to improved outcomes in subsequent disaster response. Researchers need to do a better job collectively of sharing research successes with concrete outcomes, not just results, he said.

Another challenge, McNutt added, is that when scientists do present their findings, policy makers who either do not want to spend the money or do not want to take the action can always find a scientist who will dispute or offer a different opinion on the findings. She noted that climate change science is a prime example of this.

> We do have a consensus that we need [disaster] research, that we can focus the research on enhancing both the response to the disaster and potentially affecting the individuals affected by that very disaster.
>
> —*Charles Cairns*

Cairns opined that there is a consensus that disaster research is needed, and that the research can be focused on enhancing both the response to a disaster and impacting outcomes for the individuals affected by that disaster. Scientists need to come forward with data and sound evidence that can impact this mission in the face of programmatic funding and regulatory challenges.

CREATING CONNECTIONS BETWEEN THE RESEARCH AND PRACTICE COMMUNITIES

Herrmann noted that NACCHO hosts an annual preparedness summit, bringing together more than 2,000 local, state, and federal public health care professionals, and more recent summits have included a research forum to create connections between the research community and the practice community. Herrmann shared some of the concerns raised by both NACCHO constituents and several workshop participants about public health and researchers working together. Public health departments need to understand the value and benefit of the research to them, their agencies, and their public's health. Researchers should also ask them directly what would incentivize them to participate in this research. Public health departments need to be included in the planning process from the beginning. There is also a need to address the perceived burdens associated with the health departments' participation in disaster research and provide assurance that they will still be able to perform their primary function and responsibility during the response and recovery period (protecting the health and welfare of their communities). Budget cuts over the past few years have severely impacted the services that public health departments can offer to their communities, and researchers need to recognize the limitations and the burdens that public health departments are under, especially during public health emergencies. Public health practitioners and researchers speak different languages, Herrmann said, and can be intimidated by one another. Public health departments will be more apt to embrace research if there is an open environment that allows for all levels of questions as they try to understand what researchers want of them and why. It is also important that public health departments hear about their peers who have been successful in participating in research collaborations.

Local health departments are a community and culture in and of themselves, Herrmann concluded. Researchers need to appreciate what motivates that culture and what the departments concerns and issues are, and find ways to incentivize and show the value of collaborative research relationships.

THE ACADEMIC RESEARCH SYSTEM

Sally Phillips highlighted several challenges to disaster research that are inherent within the academic research system. That system, she said, is built on competition and rewards. The underlying premise of research in academic environments is achieving tenure, and publications are the way that we disseminate what we have done. Researchers typically take data out of communities and out of situations for the purposes of generating studies and results, but there is not a lot of putting anything back in to those communities or situations, she said. Disaster research is dirty and imperfect, it does not fit well into any one box as many pure science or clinical research projects do, and researchers have concerns about its value and potential publishing ability. Universities have tremendous resources to leverage, and she suggested that disasters provide an opportunity for students to participate in the research environment and learn about engagement with a community. She stressed that this does not mean sending students into harm's way, but rather, having them participate at a secondary level by analyzing data and feeding it back to the situation, thereby getting a real sense of the struggles of that community. This will provide these next-generation clinicians, researchers, and scientists with a tremendous perspective that most do not have, she said.

McNutt suggested that academic journals could help advance research in disasters by helping to identify appropriate experts as needed from their extensive databases of potential reviewers on an extensive array of topics. She also alerted participants to the forthcoming launch of a new American Association for the Advancement of Science open-access journal, *Science Advances* that aims to encourage interdisciplinary work and remove some of the barriers to publication.[1]

LOOKING AHEAD

Some of the panelists stressed the need to "think big" to address these complex problems and to translate research into action. Research in a disaster should be as relevant as possible to the questions that matter, Redlener said, and should be done with humility because science is not perfect, it is iterative, and there are numerous sensitivities related to data collection after disasters in certain populations. Sally Phillips reiterated an earlier statement that no single researcher, team, or discipline can address these issues alone. It is necessary to leverage the strengths of different partners, including funding partners, in order to make this feasible and accomplishable for researchers, responders, and communities across the country. Making the connection between research and outcomes is essential, panelists said. As Biddinger stated, it can help to earn the trust of communities where research is being conducted, inform future disaster planning, and secure funding, which together could complete an important part of the puzzle in creating a robust science response and a resilient nation.

[1]See http://news.sciencemag.org/people-events/2014/02/aaas-launches-open-access-journal (accessed December 18, 2014).

A

References

Aldrich, T. K., J. Gustave, C. B. Hall, H. W. Cohen, M. P. Webber, R. Zeig-Owens, K. Cosenza, V. Christodoulou, L. Glass, F. Al-Othman, M. D. Weiden, K. J. Kelly, and D. J. Prezant. 2010. Lung function in rescue workers at the World Trade Center after 7 years. *New England Journal of Medicine* 362(14):1263-1272.

Banauch, G. I., C. Hall, M. Weiden, H. W. Cohen, T. K. Aldrich, V. Christodoulou, N. Arcentales, K. J. Kelly, and D. J. Prezant. 2006. Pulmonary function after exposure to the World Trade Center collapse in the New York City Fire Department. *American Journal of Respiratory and Critical Care Medicine* 174(3):312-319.

Birnbaum, M. L., E. K. Daily, A. P. O'Rourke, and A. Loretti. 2014. Disaster Research/Evaluation Frameworks, Part 1: An overview. *Prehospital Disaster Medicine* 14:1-12.

CDC (Centers for Disease Control and Prevention). 2014. Hurricane Sandy recovery research. http://www.cdc.gov/phpr/science/hurricane_sandy_recovery_research_research.html (accessed September 3, 2014).

Chen, B. C., L. K. Shawn, N. J. Connors, K. Wheeler, N. Williams, R. S. Hoffman, T. D. Matte, and S. W. Smith. 2013. Carbon monoxide exposures in New York City following Hurricane Sandy in 2012. *Clinical Toxicology (Philadelphia, PA)* 51(9):879-885.

Cho, S. J., A. Nolan, G. C. Echevarria, S. Kwon, B. Naveed, E. Schenck, J. Tsukiji, D. J. Prezant, W. N. Rom, and M. D. Weiden. 2013. Chitotriosidase is a biomarker for the resistance to World Trade Center lung injury in New York City firefighters. *Journal of Clinical Immunology* 33(6):1134-1142.

Decker, J. A., D. G. DeBord, B. Bernard, G. S. Dotson, J. Halpin, C. J. Hines, M. Kiefer, K. Myers, E. Page, P. Schulte, and J. Snawder. 2013a. Recommendations for biomonitoring of emergency responders: Focus on occupational health investigations and occupational health research. *Military Medicine* 178(1):68-75.

Decker, J. A., M. Kiefer, D. B. Reissman, R. Funk, J. Halpin, B. Bernard, R. L. Ehrenberg, C. R. Schuler, E. Whelan, K. Myers, and J. Howard. 2013b. A decision process for determining whether to conduct responder health research following large disasters. *American Journal of Disaster Medicine* 8(1):25-33.

Fireman, E. M., Y. Lerman, E. Ganor, J. Greif, S. Fireman-Shoresh, P. J. Lioy, G. I. Banauch, M. Weiden, K. J. Kelly, and D. J. Prezant. 2004. Induced sputum assessment in New York City firefighters exposed to World Trade Center dust. *Environmental Health Perspectives* 112(15):1564-1569.

IOM (Institute of Medicine). 2010. *Assessing the effects of the Gulf of Mexico oil spill on human health: Workshop summary*. Washington, DC: The National Academies Press.

Kim, H. K., M. Takematsu, R. Biary, N. Williams, R. S. Hoffman, and S. W. Smith. 2013. Epidemic gasoline exposures following Hurricane Sandy. *Prehospital Disaster Medicine* 28(6):586-591.

King, B. S., and J. D. Gibbons. 2011. Health hazard evaluation of Deepwater Horizon response workers. http://www.cdc.gov/niosh/hhe/reports/pdfs/2010-0115-0129-3138.pdf (accessed July 10, 2014).

Kitt, M. M., J. A. Decker, L. Delaney, R. Funk, J. Halpin, A. Tepper, J. Spahr, and J. Howard. 2012. Protecting workers in large-scale emergency responses: NIOSH experience in the Deepwater Horizon response. *Journal of Occupational and Environmental Medicine* 53(7):711-718.

Laskowski, L. K., G. Cruz, and S. W. Smith. 2013. Emergent communication networks during disaster: An app for that. *Disaster Medicine and Public Health Preparedness* 7(4):346-347.

Lurie, N., T. Manolio, A. P. Patterson, F. Collins, and T. Frieden. 2013. Research as a part of public health emergency response. *New England Journal of Medicine* 368(13):1251-1255.

Michaels, D., and J. Howard. 2012. Review of the OSHA-NIOSH response to the Deepwater Horizon oil spill: Protecting the health and safety of cleanup workers. *PLoS Currents: Disasters.* http://currents.plos.org/disasters?s=Deepwater+Horizon (accessed July 10, 2014).

National Institute for Occupational Safety and Health. 2011. Lessons Learned from the Deepwater Horizon Response. http://www.cdc.gov/niosh/docs/2012-117 (accessed July 10, 2014).

Nolan, A., B. Naveed, A. L. Comfort, N. Ferrier, C. B. Hall, S. Kwon, K. J. Kasturiarachchi, H. W. Cohen, R. Zeig-Owens, M. S. Glaser, M. P. Webber, T. K. Aldrich, W. N. Rom, K. Kelly, D. J. Prezant, and M. D. Weiden. 2012. Inflammatory biomarkers predict airflow obstruction after exposure to World Trade Center dust. *Chest* 142(2):412-418.

Prezant, D. J., M. Weiden, G. I. Banauch, G. McGuinness, W. N. Rom, T. K. Aldrich, and K. J. Kelly. 2002. Cough and bronchial responsiveness in firefighters at the World Trade Center site. *New England Journal of Medicine* 347(11):806-815.

Reissman, D. E., M. D. Schreiber, J. M. Shultz, and R. J. Ursano. 2009. Disaster mental and behavioral health. In *Disaster Medicine.* Edited by K. L. Koenig and C. H. Schultz. Cambridge, UK: Cambridge University Press, pp. 103-112.

Reissman, D. B., K. M. Kowalksi-Trakofler, and C. L. Katz. 2011. Public health practice and disaster resilience: A framework integrating resilience as a worker protection strategy. In *Resilience and Mental Health: Challenges Across the Lifespan,* edited by S. M. Southwick, B. T. Litz, D. Charney, and M. J. Friedman. New York: Cambridge University Press, pp. 340-358.

Schenk, E., G. Wijetunge, N. C. Mann, E. B. Lerner, A. Longthorne, and D. Dawson. 2014. Epidemiology of mass casualty incidents in the United States. *Prehospital Emergency Care* 18(3):408-416.

Tofighi, B., E. Grossman, A. R. Williams, R. Biary, J. Rotrosen, and J. D. Lee. 2014. Outcomes among buprenorphine-naloxone primary care patients after Hurricane Sandy. *Addiction Science & Clinical Practice* 9(1):3.

Zeig-Owens, R., M. P. Webber, C. B. Hall, T. Schwartz, N. Jaber, J. Weakley, T. E. Rohan, H. W. Cohen, O. Derman, T. K. Aldrich, K. Kelly, and D. J. Prezant. 2011. Early assessment of cancer outcomes in New York City firefighters after the 9/11 attacks: An observational cohort study. *Lancet* 378(9794):898-905.

B

Acronyms

ASPR	Office of the Assistant Secretary for Preparedness and Response
CASPER	Community Assessment for Public Health Emergency Response
CDC	U.S. Centers for Disease Control and Prevention
CMS	Centers for Medicare & Medicaid Services
CRS	Congressional Research Service
CSTE	Council of State and Territorial Epidemiologists
Disaster-PAST	Disaster Psychosocial Assessment and Surveillance Toolkit
DOI	U.S. Department of the Interior
DR2	National Institutes of Health Disaster Research Response Project
DSHS	Department of State Health Services–Texas
EHR	electronic health record
EMS	emergency medical services
EMT	emergency medical technician
EPA	U.S. Environmental Protection Agency
EPCR	electronic patient care report
ERHMS	Emergency Responder Health Monitoring and Surveillance System
ESF	Emergency Support Function

FACA	Federal Advisory Committee Act
FDA	U.S. Food and Drug Administration
FDNY	Fire Department of the City of New York
FEMA	Federal Emergency Management Agency
GuLF	Gulf Long-term Follow-up Study
HHS	U.S. Department of Health and Human Services
HIPAA	Health Insurance Portability and Accountability Act
ICS	incident command structure
IOM	Institute of Medicine
IRB	institutional review board
NACCHO	National Association of County and City Health Officials
NAS	National Academy of Sciences
NCEH	National Center for Environmental Health (CDC)
NDLON	National Day Laborer Organizing Network
NEMSIS	National EMS Information System
NGO	nongovernmental organization
NHTSA	National Highway Transportation Safety Administration
NIEHS	National Institute of Environmental Health Sciences
NIH	National Institutes of Health
NIMH	National Institute of Mental Health
NIOSH	National Institute for Occupational Safety and Health (CDC)
NLM	National Library of Medicine
NPRSB	National Preparedness and Research Science Board
NSF	National Science Foundation
NYAM	New York Academy of Medicine
NYU	New York University
OHSRP	Office of Human Subjects Research Protections (NIH)
OMB	Office of Management and Budget
OSHA	Occupational Safety and Health Administration
PHERRB	Public Health Emergency Research Review Board
PREP	Program for Emergency Preparedness (USCIITG)
RAPID	Grants for Rapid Response Research program (NSF)

SSG	Strategic Sciences Group (DOI)
USCIITG	U.S. Critical Illness and Injury Trials Group
UTMB	University of Texas Medical Branch
WETP	Worker Education and Training Program (NIEHS)
WTC	World Trade Center

C

Agenda

June 12, 2014
Natcher Conference Center
Masur Auditorium
Irvine, CA

1:00 p.m. **Welcome and Introductions**

AUBREY MILLER
Senior Medical Advisor
National Institute of Environmental Health Sciences, National Institutes of Health

1:15 p.m. **Moving Forward: Implementing a Research Agenda in Disasters**

NICOLE LURIE
Assistant Secretary for Preparedness and Response, Department of Health and Human Services

2:00 p.m. **Plenary Session: Overview of Case Studies Demonstrating Health Research Needs, Actions, and Lessons Learned**

Goal: Explore past research responses, needs, and priority issues of concern for framing the workshop sessions and discussions.

Overview and Introductions/Facilitator
BOB URSANO, Director, Center for the Study of Traumatic Stress, Uniformed Services University of the Health Sciences

Lessons from Katrina
DAVID ABRAMSON, Deputy Director, National Center for Disaster Preparedness at Columbia University

Research Following September 11, 2001
DAVID PREZANT, Chief Medical Officer of the Fire Department of the City of New York

Hurricane Sandy
LEWIS GOLDFRANK, Professor, Department of Emergency Medicine at New York University

4:45 p.m. **Concluding Remarks**

DONALD A. B. LINDBERG
Director, National Library of Medicine, National Institutes of Health

June 13, 2014
Natcher Conference Center
Main Auditorium
Irvine, CA

Plenary Session 2: Morning Speakers

Goal: Identifying data gaps in disasters and implementing research looking forward.

FRANCIS COLLINS
Director
National Institutes of Health

LINDA BIRNBAUM
Director
National Institute of Environmental Health Sciences

JOHN HOWARD
Director
National Institute for Occupational Safety and Health, Centers for Disease Control and Prevention

Morning Concurrent Panel Sessions

PANEL 1: ADDRESSING INSTITUTIONAL REVIEW BOARD BARRIERS TO HEALTH RESEARCH IMPLEMENTATION

Facilitator:
DIANE DIEULIIS, Deputy Director, Office of Policy and Planning, Assistant Secretary of Preparedness and Response

Goals: Explore strategies to balance human subject protections while enabling timely IRB review of research protocols, discuss strategies to obtain informed consent in emergency situations, and consider the ethics of data collection for special populations in disasters.

1. MICHAEL GOTTESMAN, Deputy Director for Intramural Research, National Institutes of Health
2. NELL ALLBRITTON, IRB Director, Louisiana Department of Health and Hospitals
3. HOLLY TAYLOR, Core Faculty, Johns Hopkins Berman Institute of Bioethics

PANEL 2: PARTNERING WITH THE COMMUNITY TO ENABLE ACCESS AND BASELINE DATA

Facilitators:
JOSEPH "CHIP" HUGHES, Program Director, Worker Education and Training Branch, NIEHS

JACK HERRMANN, Senior Advisor & Chief, Public Health Programs, NACCHO

Goals: Explore how to effectively engage community and citizen scientists in disaster research. Consider strategies to strengthen the interface and collaborations with first responders and emergency management, health departments, workers, and others to promote successful disaster research.

1. DAVID LAKEY, Commissioner, Texas Department of State Health Services
2. STEPHEN BRADBERRY, Executive Director, Alliance Institute
3. CRAIG SLATIN, Principal Investigator and Director of The New England Consortium
4. ANTHONY SPEIER, Associate Professor of Clinical Psychiatry, Louisiana State University Health Sciences Center

PANEL 3: IMPROVING DATA COLLECTION CAPABILITIES AND INFORMATION RESOURCES

Facilitator:
STEVEN PHILLIPS, National Library of Medicine, NIH

Goals: Explore new data collection tools and strategies, infrastructure needs to enable effective and accessible data sharing, and field implementation.

1. AUBREY MILLER, Senior Medical Advisor, NIEHS
2. MICHAEL HEUMANN, Oregon Public Health, Council of State and Territorial Epidemiologists

3. GAMUNU WIJETUNGE AND ELLEN SCHENK, NHTSA
4. LAUREN LEWIS, Chief of Health Studies Branch, National Center for Environmental Health (NCEH/CDC)

Lunch

Afternoon Concurrent Panel Sessions

PANEL 4: CONSIDERATIONS FOR RAPID AND SUSTAINED FUNDING MECHANISMS FOR RESEARCH IN DISASTERS

Facilitator:
GWEN COLLMAN, Director, Division of Extramural Research and Training, NIEHS

Goals: Consider rapid funding mechanisms to enable nimble and flexible grant distribution. Discuss strategies for designing funding mechanisms that would allow for sustainable disaster research protocols, which have the flexibility to immediately activate additional protocols during a disaster.

1. DENNIS WENGER, Program Director, Infrastructure Systems Management and Extreme Events, National Science Foundation
2. FAITH MITCHELL, President and CEO, Grantmakers In Health
3. SARAH LISTER, Specialist in Public Health and Epidemiology, Congressional Research Service

PANEL 5: IMPROVING THE ROLE OF EXTRAMURAL CLINICAL AND ACADEMIC RESEARCHERS, CENTERS, AND NETWORKS

Facilitator:
DAVID ABRAMSON, Deputy Director, National Center for Disaster Preparedness

Goals: Explore the essential role for the academic and clinical research community and other partners in collecting data, data sharing, communications, and other priorities to enable timely research. Discuss multiple institutions working together as one entity, and the characteristics of an ongoing, sustained research network.

1. LORI PEEK, Codirector, Center for Disaster and Risk Analysis, Colorado State University
2. GARY MACHLIS, Colead of Strategic Sciences Group, U.S. Department of the Interior
3. PAUL SELIGMAN, Executive Director, Global Regulatory Policy, Amgen
4. SHARON CROISANT, Associate Professor, Community Outreach and Education Program of the NIEHS Center in Environmental Toxicology, University of Texas Medical Branch (UTMB)

Panel 6: Coordinating Logistics to Execute Rapid Research in Disaster Response

Facilitator:
HOWARD ZUCKER, Acting Commissioner, New York State Department of Health

Goals: Discuss triggers for go/no-go scenarios, just-in-time training for research responders, integration of disaster research response into the ICS structure, and corresponding logistical needs when working in disaster settings.

1. SHELLEY DUTEAUX, Assistant Deputy Director of Public Health Emergency Preparedness, California Department of Public Health
2. CHARLES CAIRNS, Associate Director, U.S. Critical Illness and Injury Trials Group
3. JOSEPH "CHIP" HUGHES, Program Director, Worker Education and Training Branch, NIEHS
4. JOSEPH BARBERA, CoDirector of the Institute for Crisis, Disaster and Risk Management at George Washington University

Break

Plenary Session 3: Wrap Up and Next Steps
Main Auditorium

Goals: Provide bold strategies for improved inclusion and integration of all stakeholders to support the timely identification of health research priorities, and collection of longer-term data to understand health impacts, efficacy of responses, and risk factors to strengthen resiliency and future preparedness.

REPORT BACK FROM PANEL DISCUSSIONS

Goal: Top 5 action items from each category for a 5-year horizon to improve our health research response capabilities

CLOSING RESPONSE PANEL: ACTIONS TO BUILD THE FUTURE FOR DISASTER RESEARCH

Facilitator:
BERNARD GOLDSTEIN, Emeritus Professor and Dean, University of Pittsburgh Graduate School of Public Health

1. MARCIA MCNUTT, Editor-in-Chief, *Science*
2. JACK HERRMANN, Senior Advisor and Chief, Public Health Programs, NACCHO
3. IRWIN REDLENER, Director, National Center for Disaster Preparedness
4. SALLY PHILLIPS, Acting Deputy Assistant Secretary, Office of Health Affairs, DHS
5. PAUL BIDDINGER, Medical Director for Emergency Preparedness, Massachusetts General Hospital and Partners Healthcare

D

Biographical Sketches of Invited Speakers and Panelists

David Abramson, Ph.D., M.P.H., is Deputy Director and Director of Research at Columbia University's National Center for Disaster Preparedness at the Earth Institute. Dr. Abramson's areas of interest include disaster recovery and resiliency, the social ecology of vulnerability, risk communication targeted at high-risk or elusive communities, and rapid research strategies in postdisaster settings. Dr. Abramson is the principal investigator of the longitudinal Gulf Coast Child & Family Health Study, an examination of need and recovery among 1,000+ randomly sampled displaced and impacted families in Louisiana and Mississippi (2006–2010), and is Coinvestigator of an National Institutes of Health (NIH) study of the impact of the Deepwater Horizon oil spill on children's health. Additionally, Dr. Abramson is leading a foundation-funded effort to identify pediatric need along the Gulf Coast coupled with a youth empowerment intervention project in five Gulf Coast high schools. Other current or recent disaster-related research activities include studies of how U.S. cities recover from disasters, evolving trends in disaster philanthropy, the public health response to Hurricanes Irene and Sandy, and the facilitation of health care coalitions in New York City. Prior to entering the field of public health in 1990, Dr. Abramson worked for a decade as a national magazine journalist, having written for *Rolling Stone, Esquire, Outside,* and the *San Francisco Examiner*, among other publications. A former paramedic, Abramson holds a doctorate in sociomedical sciences with a specialization in political science and a master of public health degree, both from Columbia University.

Nell W. Allbritton, M.P.A., leads the institutional review board (IRB) for the Louisiana Department of Health and Hospitals (DHH) as the Director and Interim Chair. At DHH, she spearheads the reinvigoration of the DHH IRB to meet national best practices, maximizing the impact of research on Louisiana's public health while protecting DHH consumers as human participants. As the DHH Data Compliance Officer, Ms. Allbritton also ensures DHH's sharing of data meets federal and state regulatory requirements. She has been active in government administration at the federal, state, and local levels for 15 years, most recently as staff to New Orleans Mayor Mitchell J. Landrieu. She began her M.P.A. at George Washington University in Washington, DC, and graduated with her M.P.A. from the E.J. Ourso College of Business at Louisiana State University in Baton Rouge.

Joseph A. Barbera, M.D., is CoDirector of the George Washington University (GWU) Institute for Crisis, Disaster, and Risk Management (ICDRM) (www.gwu.edu/~icdrm) in Washington, DC. He is also an Associate Professor of Engineering Management and Clinical Associate Professor of Emergency Medicine at GWU, where he created and teaches Masters and Doctoral level academic courses in emergency management. He has enjoyed a 25-year career as an emergency responder and consultant on emergency management. He was the lead medical consultant for the Federal Emergency Management Agency (FEMA) in the development of the National Urban Search & Rescue (US&R) Response System, and performed the same role for the Office of U.S. Foreign Disaster Assistance (OFDA) in developing the International Search & Rescue program. As member of the Fairfax County (Virginia) US&R Task Force, he participates as a medical officer for OFDA and FEMA responses and for the FEMA US&R Incident Support Team. His experience includes on-scene-response to hurricanes (2005 Hurricanes Katrina and Wilma and others), mine disasters, earthquakes (Baguio City Philippines 1990, Northridge California 1994, Tou-Liu Taiwan 1999, and Haiti 2010), terrorist incidents (the Oklahoma City Bombing and the 9-11 Pentagon and World Trade Center attacks), bio-terrorism (Anthrax 2001), tsunami (Banda Aceh, Indonesia), and school collapse (Haiti 2008). He has helped plan and execute medical contingency capabilities for high security events (presidential inaugurations, State of the Union addresses, the North Atlantic Treaty Organization's 50th Anniversary Summit). As founding chair of the D.C. Hospital Association Emergency Preparedness Committee, Dr. Barbera coordinated the implementation of the Hospital Mutual Aid System for Washington, DC.

He has completed multiple research projects focusing on health and medical systems in emergency response and published a range of articles and guidance documents for emergency management and emergency response.

Georges C. Benjamin, M.D., FACP, FACEP(E), FNAPA, Hon FRSPH, is the Executive Director of the American Public Health Association (APHA), the nation's oldest and largest organization of public health professionals. He was secretary of the Maryland Department of Health and Mental Hygiene from 1999 to 2002, following 4 years as its Deputy Secretary for public health services. For 20 years he has been actively practicing public health at the local, state, and national levels with expertise in the areas of emergency preparedness, administration and infectious diseases. Dr. Benjamin serves as publisher of the field's premier journal, the *American Journal of Public Health*, The Nation's Health Newspaper and the APHA's timeless publication on infectious diseases, the *Control of Communicable Diseases Manual.* He is the author of more than 100 scientific articles and book chapters. His recent book, *The Quest for Health Reform: A Satirical History,* is an exposé of the nearly 100-year quest to ensure quality affordable health coverage for all through the use of political cartoons. Dr. Benjamin is a graduate of the Illinois Institute of Technology and the University of Illinois College of Medicine. He is board certified in internal medicine and a Fellow of the American College of Physicians; he also is a Fellow emeritus of the American College of Emergency Physicians, an honorary Fellow of the Royal Society of Public Health, a Fellow of the National Academy of Public Administration, and a member of the Institute of Medicine (IOM) of the National Academies.

Paul Biddinger, M.D., FACEP, is the Vice Chairman for Emergency Preparedness in the Department of Emergency Medicine at Massachusetts General Hospital (MGH) in Boston. He is also the Medical Director for Emergency Preparedness at MGH and at Partners Healthcare. Dr. Biddinger additionally serves as the Director of the Emergency Preparedness and Response Exercise Program (EPREP) at the Harvard School of Public Health and holds appointments at Harvard Medical School and at the Harvard School of Public Health. He chairs the Massachusetts Medical Society's Committee on Preparedness and serves as a medical officer for the MA-1 Disaster Medical Assistance Team (DMAT) in the National Disaster Medical System (NDMS) in the U.S. Department of Health and Human Services (HHS). He is an active researcher in the field of emergency preparedness and has lectured nationally and internationally on topics of preparedness and disaster medicine. He has authored numerous articles and book chapters on multiple topics related to emergency medical services and disaster medicine. He completed his undergraduate study in international relations at Princeton University, attended medical school at Vanderbilt University, and completed residency training in emergency medicine at Harvard.

Linda Birnbaum, Ph.D., DABT, ATS, became the Director of the National Institute of Environmental Health Sciences (NIEHS), NIH, and the National Toxicology Program (NTP) on January 18, 2009. In these roles Dr. Birnbaum oversees federal funding for biomedical research to discover how the environment influences human health and disease. Several advisory boards and councils provide Dr. Birnbaum and NIEHS/NTP staff with input to accomplish this large task. Dr. Birnbaum is the first toxicologist and the first woman to lead the NIEHS/NTP. She has spent most of her career as a federal scientist. She has received numerous awards and recognitions, including being elected to the Institute of Medicine (IOM) of the National Academies in October 2010, one of the highest honors in the fields of medicine and health. Dr. Birnbaum's own research and many of her publications focus on the pharmacokinetic behavior of environmental chemicals; mechanisms of actions of toxicants, including endocrine disruption; and linking of real-world exposures to health effects. Dr. Birnbaum also finds time to mentor the next generation of environmental health scientists. For example, she serves as adjunct professor in the Gillings School of Global Public Health, the Curriculum in Toxicology, and the Department of Environmental Sciences and Engineering at the University of North Carolina at Chapel Hill, as well as in the Integrated Toxicology Program at Duke University. A native of New Jersey, Dr. Birnbaum received her M.S. and Ph.D. in microbiology from the University of Illinois at Urbana-Champaign.

Stephen Bradberry, B.S., is the Executive Director of Alliance Institute, the Gulf South's premier nonprofit organization for training and technical skills assistance to individuals, communities, and organizations seeking to increase their capacity for community engagement. The organization currently oversees the community involvement portion of the Gulf Region Health Outreach Program, a 5-year program to strengthen health care, health literacy, and resiliency of Gulf Coast communities affected by the BP oil drilling disaster. A Chicago native, Mr. Bradberry is a veteran community organizer who has worked with low- and moderate-income families and individuals for more than 20 years. His work has centered on organizing public interest campaigns to actively involve low-income families in addressing the social problems they face. He has led campaigns promoting a living wage, preventing predatory lending, preventing lead poisoning in children, and increasing voter participation. He has been tapped by the Robert F. Kennedy Foundation of Europe to assist in the development of their Human Rights Training Institute and mentors young activists, advocates, and organizers across the United States. In 2005, Mrs. Ethel Kennedy and Senator Edward Kennedy presented Bradberry with the Robert F. Kennedy Human Rights Award for his efforts on behalf of the poor. At the event, then-Senator Barack Obama congratulated Mr. Bradberry for his work to defend the rights of the poor in New Orleans, saying, "You deserve this day in the sun," and noting that Mr. Bradberry's social activism plays to Robert Kennedy's vision of a better world: "Somewhere there's always been people like Steve Bradberry who believe that this isn't the way it's supposed to be. People who believe that while evil and suffering will always exist, this is a country that has been fueled by small miracles and boundless dreams."

Charles B. Cairns, M.D., FACEP, FAAEM, FAHA, is Professor and Chair of the Department of Emergency Medicine at the University of North Carolina at Chapel Hill. He previously served as the Director of Emergency Research at the Duke Clinical Research Institute (2004–2008), the largest academic clinical research organization in the world. For the past 25 years, Dr. Cairns has been a clinician, educator, investigator, and leader in emergency care focused on optimization of the host responses of individual patients and populations to acute and emergency medical conditions. His efforts have positively impacted the host response to infection, ischemia, injury and resuscitation for applications in emergency patient care, health systems and preparedness at the local, state, and national levels. He is currently the Principal Investigator (PI) of the U.S. Department of Homeland Security's (DHS) National Biosurveillance Integration Center (NBIC) National Collaborative for Bio-preparedness, and the Associate Director of the NIH U.S. Critical Illness and Injury Trials Group. Dr. Cairns has published more than 150 scientific articles and reviews, and he has received numerous awards and honors, including the Emergency Medicine Foundation (EMF) Career Development Award, the EMF Established Investigator Award, the American College of Emergency Physicians (ACEP) Outstanding Contribution in Research Award, and the 2014 John Marx Leadership Award, the highest award of the Society for Academic

Emergency Medicine (SAEM). Dr. Cairns has served in leadership positions within organized emergency medicine, including Co-Chair of the ACEP-SAEM Research Working Group, SAEM Program Chair, ACEP Research Committee Chair, and ACEP Scientific Review Committee Chair, and member of the EMF Board of Trustees, the Leadership Committee for the American Heart Association (AHA) Council on Cardiopulmonary and Critical Care, the Steering Committee for the Critical Care Societies Collaborative (CCSC) Task Force on Critical Care Research, and the Coordination Committee for the NIH National Asthma Education and Prevention Program. He was also a Co-Chair of the NIH Roundtables on Emergency Research. He has served on the editorial boards of both *Academic Emergency Medicine* and the *Annals of Emergency Medicine*. Dr. Cairns is an honors graduate of Dartmouth College and was a Holderness Medical Fellow at the University of North Carolina, where he received the Medical Faculty Award as the outstanding graduating medical student. He completed an emergency medicine residency and EMF Research Fellowship at the Harbor UCLA Medical Center. After serving on the UCLA faculty, he moved to the University of Colorado, where he became Director of the Colorado Emergency Medicine Research Center, leading it to become one of the first three national EMF Centers of Excellence. Dr. Cairns is board certified in emergency medicine, a Fellow of the American College of Emergency Physicians, and a Fellow of the American Heart Association.

Gwen Collman, Ph.D., is Director of the NIEHS Division of Extramural Research and Training, where she leads approximately 70 professional staff in areas of scientific program administration, peer review, and the management and administration of about 1,500 active grants each year. She directs scientific activities across the field of environmental health sciences, including basic sciences (i.e., DNA repair, epigenetics), organ-specific toxicology (i.e., reproductive, respiratory), public health–related programs (i.e., environmental epidemiology and public health), and training and career development. She also oversees the implementation of the Superfund Research Program, the Worker Education and Training Program, and the NIEHS Centers for Nanotechnology Health Implications Research consortium. Prior to her current role, Dr. Collman served in program development and management, beginning in 1992 and as Chief of the Susceptibility and Population Health Branch. During this time, she directed research on the role of genetic and environmental factors on the development of human disease, from animal models of genetic susceptibility to population studies focusing on etiology and intervention. She was responsible for building the NIEHS grant portfolio in environmental and molecular epidemiology and developed several complex multi-disciplinary research programs. These include the NIEHS Breast Cancer and the Environment Research Centers Program, the NIEHS/Environmental Protection Agency Centers for Children's Environmental Health and Disease Prevention, and the Genes, Environment and Health Initiative. Also, under her guidance a team created a vision for the Partnerships for Environmental Public Health programs. Dr. Collman received a Ph.D. in environmental epidemiology from University of North Carolina School of Public Health in 1984.

Sharon Croisant (Petronella), Ph.D., M.S., is an Associate Professor on the faculty of the School of Medicine's Department of Preventive Medicine and Community Health. She holds a doctorate in epidemiology and a master's in health promotion and education. She also currently directs the NIEHS-funded University of Texas Medical Branch Center in Environmental Toxicology's Community-based Research Facility as well as its Community Outreach and Engagement Core. She is a Center investigator within the Institute for Translational Sciences, which houses the University's Clinical and Translational Science Award, for which she serves as Director of the Community Engagement and Research Key Resource. A major focus of her career has been translational or integrative research, i.e., building interfaces between and among environmental and clinical research, education, and community health. She has considerable expertise in Community-Based Participatory Research, including its applications in Environmental Justice communities, and is currently the co-PI of a grant from NIEHS to investigate the long-term health effects of consumption of Gulf seafood potentially contaminated by the explosion of the Deepwater Horizon and the resulting unprecedented oil spill. She has collaborated on multiple projects designed to elucidate the causes and mechanisms of asthma exacerbations related to air pollution and has established long-standing, ongoing collaborative relationships with community stakeholders with a vested interest in using these research findings to direct community-based intervention and outreach activities. An active member of the UTMB faculty, she is the past Chair of the institutional Faculty Senate and serves on a national Scientific Advisory Panel for the Environmental Protection Agency. She is now in the process of developing a more fully integrated Gulf Coast Regional Environmental Health Science Network, building on relationships previously established with coastal communities in the aftermath of both natural and man-made disasters.

Diane DiEuliis, Ph.D., is the Deputy Director for Policy in the Office of the Assistant Secretary for Preparedness and Response (ASPR), HHS, a position she has held since August 2011. In this position, she is responsible for assisting in the coordination of policy and strategic planning for components of ASPR and directly supporting the Deputy Assistant Secretary for Policy. Prior to joining HHS, Dr. DiEuliis was the Assistant Director for Life Sciences and Behavioral and Social Sciences in the Office of Science and Technology Policy (OSTP) in the Executive Office of the President. During her 4-year tenure at the White House, she was responsible for coordinating health issues among federal departments and agencies and was involved in developing policy in areas such as biosecurity, biosafety, human subjects, synthetic biology, federal scientific collections, public access, and biotechnology. She also managed portfolios in the Science of Science Policy (devoted to measuring the outcomes of federal investments in science and technology), and Research Business Models (devoted to streamlining administrative requirements in the grants and contracts process). Dr. DiEuliis also worked to help coordinate agency response to public health issues such as the H1N1 flu. Prior to working at OSTP, she was a Program Director at NIH, where she managed a diverse portfolio of neuroscience research in neurodegenerative diseases such as Alzheimer's and Parkinson's. She completed a fellowship at the University of Pennsylvania in the Center for Neurodegenerative Disease Research. She obtained her Ph.D. degree from the University of Delaware and completed her postdoctoral research in the NIH Intramural research program, where she focused on cellular and molecular neuroscience.

Shelley DuTeaux, Ph.D., M.P.H., is the Assistant Deputy Director for Public Health Emergency Preparedness for the California Department of Public Health (CDPH). Prior to joining CDPH, Dr. DuTeaux was the Emergency Response Coordinator for the California Air Resources Board, where she assisted with monitoring, modeling, and assessing toxic air releases. She also served as lead toxicologist for the California Accidental Release Prevention Program and as the Emergency Response Coordinator for the California Office of Environmental Health Hazard Assessment. Before coming to work for the state of California in 2005, Dr. DuTeaux held multiple positions at the national weapons laboratories, with the state of New Mexico, and with nonprofit health agencies. Dr. DuTeaux is a recognized expert in exposure assessment of wildfire smoke and has presented extensively on the subject. She is also the immediate past Chair of the California Air Response Planning Alliance. Dr. DuTeaux holds a master's in public health (UC Berkeley) and a Ph.D. in pharmacology and toxicology (UC Davis) and is a certified Hazardous Materials Technical Reference Specialist (Title 29 CCR 1910.120).

Lewis R. Goldfrank, M.D. (IOM), has worked at Bellevue Hospital Center and New York University (NYU) Medical Center for 30 years. He is currently the first Chairman and Professor of the newly established academic Department of Emergency Medicine at NYU, where his efforts have led to the development of the university's emergency medicine and medical toxicology residencies. Dr. Goldfrank is also the Medical Director of the New York City Health Department's Poison Center. His career has been spent working in the public hospitals of New York City, emphasizing the role of emergency medicine in improving access to care, public health, public policy, and medical humanism. He has assisted in numerous projects in South America, Asia, and Europe in the advancement of emergency medicine and medical toxicology, emphasizing his interests in the improvement of global health. His current global health efforts involve the development of emergency medicine in Accra, Ghana. Dr. Goldfrank has served on three committees (as Chair for two of them) dealing with issues of terrorism: civilian medical response to chemical and biological terrorism, metropolitan medical response teams and preparedness for terrorism, and the psychological consequences of terrorism. Educated at Clark University, the Johns Hopkins School of Medicine, and the University of Brussels, Belgium, he graduated from the University of Brussels Medical School in 1970. He completed his residency in Internal Medicine at Montefiore Hospital and Medical Center in 1973. He is the senior editor of *Goldfrank's Toxicologic Emergencies,* a standard text in the field now in its 10th edition. He is a member of the IOM.

Bernard D. Goldstein, M.D., is Emeritus Professor of Environmental and Occupational Health and former dean of the University of Pittsburgh Graduate School of Public Health. He is a physician, board certified in internal medicine, hematology, and in toxicology. Dr. Goldstein is author of more than 150 publications in the peer-reviewed literature, as well as numerous reviews related to environmental health. He is an elected member of the National Academy of Sciences (NAS) IOM and of the American Society for Clinical Investigation. His experience includes service as Assistant Administrator for Research and Development of the EPA, 1983–1985. In 2001 he came to the University of Pittsburgh from New Jersey, where he had been the Founding Director of the Environmental and

Occupational Health Sciences Institute, a joint program of Rutgers University and Robert Wood Johnson Medical School. He has chaired more than a dozen National Research Council and IOM committees primarily related to environmental health issues. He has been President of the Society for Risk Analysis, and has chaired the NIH Toxicology Study Section, EPA's Clean Air Scientific Advisory Committee, the National Board of Public Health Examiners, and the Research Committee of the Health Effects Institute. He has also served as a member or chairperson of numerous national and international scientific advisory committees for government, industry, and environmental groups.

Michael Gottesman, M.D., has been Deputy Director for Intramural Research at NIH since 1993. A graduate of Harvard College and Harvard Medical School, Dr. Gottesman completed an internship and residency at the Peter Bent Brigham Hospital in Boston. He was a research associate at NIH from 1971 to 1974. He returned to Harvard Medical School as an Assistant Professor before returning to NIH in 1976. Dr. Gottesman became Chief of the Laboratory of Cell Biology in the National Cancer Institute in 1990. From 1992 to 1993, he was Acting Director for the National Center for Human Genome Research (NCHGR), and he was Acting Scientific Director of NCHGR in 1993. His research interests have ranged from how DNA is replicated in bacteria to how cancer cells elude chemotherapy. He has published extensively on these subjects, with more than 400 scientific publications to his credit. He has helped to identify the human gene that causes cancer cells to resist many anticancer drugs. He has shown that this gene encodes a protein that pumps anticancer drugs out of drug-resistant human cancers and has used this information to create gene transfer vectors and to circumvent drug resistance in cancer. He has been a member of the IOM since 2003 and the American Academy of Arts and Sciences since 2009. Dr. Gottesman has been actively involved in initiating several training and mentoring programs for high school students and teachers, as well as college, medical, and graduate students. As Deputy Director for Intramural Research at NIH, he has initiated an NIH-wide lecture series and reformulated tenure and review processes in the intramural program. He has also instituted training programs for minority and disadvantaged students, loan repayment programs for clinical researchers at NIH, and a research training program for medical students.

Jack Herrmann, M.S.Ed., N.C.C., L.M.H.C., is the Senior Advisor and Chief, Public Health Programs, at the National Association of County and City Health Officials (NACCHO), an association representing the interests of the country's 2,800 local governmental public health departments. As the organization's chief liaison to local, state, and federal partner agencies, his portfolio includes public health preparedness, environmental health, infectious disease prevention and control, public health law, health and disability, and public health informatics. Mr. Herrmann is also the organization's subject-matter expert on a variety of preparedness and response topics including, mass fatalities planning, medical countermeasure distribution and dispensing, bioterrorism preparedness, and disaster mental health. Prior to joining NACCHO, Mr. Herrmann was Assistant Professor of Psychiatry and Clinical Nursing, Director of the Program in Disaster Mental Health, and Director of Community and Consumer Affairs for the University of Rochester Medical Center, Department of Psychiatry. He has served in volunteer staff or leadership positions with the American Red Cross for the past 20 years, responding to such disasters as the Northridge Earthquake, the explosion of TWA Flight 800, the terrorist events of September 11, 2001, and Hurricanes Katrina, Rita, and Sandy. Mr. Herrmann earned a master's degree in education in counseling, family, and worklife studies from the University of Rochester, is certified by the National Board of Certified Counselors (NBCC), and is a licensed mental health counselor in the state of New York.

Michael Heumann, M.P.H., M.A., has been an epidemiologist in occupational and environmental public health since 1981. From June 1984 through July 2011, he was the lead occupational and environmental epidemiologist at the Oregon Public Health Division (OPHD), Oregon Health Authority. From 2002 through 2011 he developed the occupational and environmental epidemiological approaches to public health emergency preparedness within OPHD. Beginning in 2007, Mr. Heumann worked closely with the National Institute for Occupational Safety and Health (NIOSH) and the National Center for Environmental Health, as well as with state epidemiologists across the country (through the Council of State and Territorial Epidemiologists, or CSTE) to develop disaster epidemiology as a core part of public health response to all phases of the disaster management cycle. He chaired the Disaster Epidemiology Subcommittee for CSTE from 2007 through 2011. Through CSTE he developed the National Disaster Epidemiology Workshop (now in its fifth year), which brings together experts from across the country from state, local, tribal, and federal public health agencies, from academia, and from other response agencies to deepen our understanding of and improve our capabilities to plan for, respond to, and recover from natural and manmade disasters. Mr. Heumann served as one of two state occupational health representatives on the NIOSH working group that developed the Emergency Responder Health Monitoring and Surveillance (ERHMS) framework and guidance document. He then participated as a consultant to NIOSH on the development of the in-person ERHMS training course, as well as the online, self-study course curricula for ERHMS. ERHMS is now one of three disaster epidemiology trainings that are jointly provided regionally for state and local health departments across the country. Mr. Heumann is currently a consultant to CSTE and NIOSH on disaster epidemiology. He holds a master's of public health in epidemiology from UCLA and a master's degree in Latin American Studies, also from UCLA.

John Howard, M.D., is the Director of NIOSH in HHS. Dr. Howard also serves as the Administrator of the World Trade Center (WTC) Health Program in HHS. He was first appointed NIOSH Director in 2002 during the George W. Bush administration and served in that position until 2008. In 2008 and 2009 Dr. Howard worked as a consultant with the U.S. government's Afghanistan Health Initiative. In September 2009, he was again appointed NIOSH Director in the Obama administration. Prior to his appointments as NIOSH Director, Dr. Howard served as Chief of the Division of Occupational Safety and Health in the state of California's Labor and Workforce Development Agency from 1991 through 2002. Dr. Howard received a doctor of medicine degree from Loyola University of Chicago, a master of public health degree from the Harvard School of Public Health, a doctor of law degree from UCLA, and a master of law degree in administrative law and economic regulation from George Washington University in Washington, DC. Dr. Howard is board-certified in internal medicine and occupational medicine. He is admitted to the practice of medicine and law in the state of California and in the District of Columbia, and he is a member of the U.S. Supreme Court bar. He has written numerous articles on occupational health law and policy.

Joseph "Chip" Hughes, M.P.H., is currently the Director of an innovative federal safety and health training program based at NIEHS. The program supports cooperative agreements to develop and deliver model safety and health training programs for workers involved in hazardous substances response with numerous universities, unions, community colleges, and other nonprofit organizations throughout the nation. For the past 20 years, Mr. Hughes has worked in both the private and public sectors in developing environmental and occupational health education programs for workers and citizens in high-risk occupations and communities. As a part of this work, he has pioneered efforts to create new methods and approaches for conducting needs assessments, reaching underserved populations, developing training partnerships, and creating innovative program evaluation and assessment measures. Mr. Hughes was given the HHS Secretary's Award for Exceptional Service in November 2001 for his role in responding to the WTC attacks. After the NIEHS response to the Katrina disaster, Mr. Hughes was given the HHS Secretary's Award for Distinguished Service in June 2006 and the NIH Director's Award in 2011 for responding to the Deepwater Horizon oil spill. In November 2011, Mr. Hughes was given the Tony Mazzocchi Award for lifetime achievement by the National Council for Occupational Safety and Health. Under Mr. Hughes's leadership, NIEHS grant support of $40 million is annually committed for the development and administration of model worker health and safety training programs consisting of classroom, hands-on, online, computer-based, and practical health and safety training of workers and their supervisors who are engaged in activities related to hazardous materials and emergency response.

David L. Lakey, M.D., serves as Commissioner of the Texas Department of State Health Services, leading one of the state's largest agencies with a staff of 11,500 and an annual budget of $2.5 billion. As Commissioner, Dr. Lakey oversees programs such as disease prevention and bioterrorism preparedness, family and community health services, environmental and consumer safety, regulatory programs, and mental health and substance abuse prevention and treatment programs. Dr. Lakey became Commissioner on January 2, 2007. Prior to becoming Commissioner, Dr. Lakey served as an Associate Professor of Medicine, Chief of the Division of Clinical Infectious Disease, and Medical Director of the Center for Pulmonary and Infectious Disease Control at the University of Texas (UT) Health Center in Tyler. He had been a faculty member there since 1998. At the UT Center for Biosecurity and Public Health Preparedness, Dr. Lakey served as Associate Director for Infectious Disease and Biosecurity. He also chaired a bioterrorism preparedness committee for 34 hospitals in East Texas and led the development of the Public Health Laboratory of East Texas in 2002. He earned a bachelor of science in chemistry, graduating with high honors from Rose-Hulman Institute of Technology in Terre Haute, Indiana, and received his medical degree with honors from Indiana University School of Medicine. Dr. Lakey was a resident in internal medicine and pediatric medicine and completed a fellowship in adult and pediatric infectious disease at Vanderbilt University Medical Center in Nashville, Tennessee.

CAPT Lauren Lewis, M.D., M.P.H., is currently Chief of the Health Studies Branch (HSB) within the National Center for Environmental Health (NCEH), Centers for Disease Control and Prevention (CDC). In this role, she oversees the emergency response to a variety of environmental threats including disease outbreaks and clusters related to toxic exposures as well as natural, chemical, and radiological disasters. She also directs environmental epidemiological research and programs to help international, state, and local governments build epidemiological capacity to address environmental concerns. Dr. Lewis first joined HSB in 2003 as a Medical Epidemiologist, then became Branch Chief in 2008. Her accomplishments include successfully leading responses to the diethylene glycol mass poisoning in Panama and aflatoxicosis outbreaks in Kenya. She initiated, developed, and continues to direct research programs to address aflatoxins in Africa and drinking water exposures among tribal nations in the United States. She leads the Private Well Initiative, a national research program to further the knowledge on health impacts associated with private well drinking water. In 1999 Dr. Lewis began her career in public health and came to CDC as an Epidemic Intelligence Service Officer (EISO) in the Division of Violence Prevention, National Center for Injury Prevention and Control. After completing EIS training, she earned an M.P.H. in epidemiology from Emory University. She then served as a preventive medicine resident at the Indian Health Service, National Epidemiology Program in Albuquerque, New Mexico, prior to joining HSB. Prior to her career in public health, Dr. Lewis attended Howard University, Washington, DC, where she earned her B.S. and M.D. degrees. She practiced internal medicine in Atlanta, Georgia, and served as a Clinical Instructor for Morehouse College of Medicine.

Donald A. B. Lindberg, M.D., is a scientist who has been a pioneer in applying computer technology to health care, beginning in 1960 at the University of Missouri. In 1984 he was appointed Director of the National Library of Medicine (NLM), the world's largest biomedical library (annual budget $275 million; 690 career staff). From 1992 to 1995 he served in a concurrent position as founding Director of the National Coordination Office for High Performance Computing and Communications in the Office of Science and Technology Policy, Executive Office of the President. In 1996 he was named by the HHS Secretary to be the U.S. Coordinator for the G-7 Global Health Applications Project. In addition to an eminent career in pathology, Dr. Lindberg has made notable contributions to information and computer activities in medical diagnosis, artificial intelligence, and educational programs. Before his appointment as NLM Director, he was Professor of Information Science and Professor of Pathology at the University of Missouri–Columbia. He has current academic appointments as Clinical Professor of Pathology at the University of Virginia and Adjunct Professor of Pathology at the University of Maryland School of Medicine. Dr. Lindberg was elected the first President of the American Medical Informatics Association (AMIA). As the country's senior statesman for medicine and computers, he has been called on to serve on many boards, including the Computer Science and Engineering Board of the NAS, the National Board of Medical Examiners, and the Council of the IOM of the National Academy of Sciences. Dr. Lindberg graduated magna cum laude from Amherst College and received his M.D. degree from the College of Physicians and Surgeons, Columbia University.

Sarah A. Lister, D.V.M., M.P.H., is a specialist in public health and epidemiology with the Congressional Research Service, a federal legislative branch support agency. She came to Capitol Hill as an American Association for the Advancement of Science Congressional Science Fellow in 1997, sponsored by the American Veterinary Medical Association, and worked on food safety issues for the Senate Committee on Agriculture. She has served as a commissioned officer in the U.S. Public Health Service, working for CDC and for the U.S. Department of Agriculture Food Safety and Inspection Service. In addition, she has worked on issues of public health infrastructure and emergency preparedness for two public health professional associations in Washington, DC. Dr. Lister began her career as a practicing veterinarian. She holds B.S. and doctor of veterinary medicine degrees from Cornell University and a master's degree in public health from the Johns Hopkins Bloomberg School of Public Health. She is board certified in veterinary preventive medicine.

Nicole Lurie, M.D., M.S.P.H., is Assistant Secretary for Preparedness and Response (ASPR) at HHS. The ASPR serves as the Secretary's principal advisor on matters related to bioterrorism and other public health emergencies. The mission of her office is to lead the nation in preventing, responding to and recovering from the adverse health effects of public health emergencies and disasters. As such, she coordinates interagency activities among HHS, other federal agencies, and state and local officials responsible for emergency preparedness and the protection of the civilian population from acts of bioterrorism and other public health emergencies. Previously, Dr. Lurie was Senior Natural Scientist and the Paul O'Neill Alcoa Professor of Health Policy at the RAND Corporation, where she directed RAND's public health and preparedness work as well as its Center for Population Health and Health Disparities. Prior to that she served as Principal Deputy Assistant Secretary of Health for HHS; in state government as Medical Advisor to the Commissioner at the Minnesota Department of Health; and in academia as Professor in the University of Minnesota Schools of Medicine and Public Health. Dr. Lurie has a long history in the health services research field, primarily in the areas of access to and quality of care, mental health, prevention, public health infrastructure and preparedness, and health disparities. She attended college and medical school at the University of Pennsylvania, and completed her residency and M.S.P.H. at UCLA, where she was also a Robert Wood Johnson Foundation Clinical Scholar. She served as Senior Editor for *Health Services Research* and as President of the Society of General Internal Medicine, as well as on numerous other national committees. She is the recipient of many awards and is a member of the IOM. Finally, Dr. Lurie continues to practice clinical medicine in the health care safety net in Washington, DC.

Gary Machlis, Ph.D., is Science Advisor to the Director, National Park Service, and Coleader of the Strategic Sciences Group (SSG) of the Department of the Interior. He is also Professor of Environmental Sustainability at Clemson University. Dr. Machlis is the first scientist to serve in the position of Science Advisor to the Director and helped co-found the SSG in response to the Deepwater Horizon oil spill. His research focuses on science during crisis, conservation, and warfare ecology—applying ecology to issues of war preparation, violent conflict, and humanitarian and restoration response. Dr. Machlis has worked in China (on the Giant Panda Project), the Galapagos Islands, Haiti (after the earthquake), Cuba, Africa, and elsewhere. In 2010 he was elected a Fellow of the AAAS.

Marcia McNutt, Ph.D., is a geophysicist who became the 19th Editor-in-Chief of *Science* in June 2013. From 2009 to 2013, Dr. McNutt was the Director of the U.S. Geological Survey, which responded to a number of major disasters during her tenure, including the Deepwater Horizon oil spill. For her work to help contain that spill, Dr. McNutt was awarded the U.S.

Coast Guard's Meritorious Service Medal. She is a Fellow of American Geophysical Union, the Geological Society of America, AAAS, and the International Association of Geodesy. Her honors and awards include membership in the NAS, the American Philosophical Society, and the American Academy of Arts and Sciences, as well as honorary doctoral degrees from Colorado College, the University of Minnesota, Monmouth University, and the Colorado School of Mines. Dr. McNutt was awarded the Macelwane Medal by AGU in 1988 for research accomplishments by a young scientist and the Maurice Ewing Medal in 2007 for her significant contributions to deep-sea exploration.

Aubrey Miller, M.D., M.P.H., joined the NIEHS team in May 2010 to serve as Senior Medical Advisor and NIEHS liaison to HHS. Dr. Miller's office is located on the NIH campus in Bethesda, where he oversees a small staff of NIEHS employees who are readily available to meet with NIH and HHS representatives, federal partners, members of Congress, and other stakeholders to discuss how environmental factors influence human health and disease. Dr. Miller is coordinating many federal efforts, including playing a major role in NIEHS and HHS response to the Gulf of Mexico oil spill. A medical epidemiologist and a Captain in USPHS, Dr. Miller has long-standing experience, publications, and contributions to a wide range of occupational and environmental health issues and policies. Dr. Miller previously served as the Chief Medical Officer for the U.S. Food and Drug Administration (FDA), Office of Counterterrorism and Emerging Threats. Previously he worked as a Senior Medical Officer and Regional Toxicologist for EPA and for the HHS Office of the Secretary in Denver, providing leadership, expertise, and coordination for multi-agency emergency responses, such as the Libby Montana asbestos situation, the anthrax attacks in Washington, DC, and Hurricane Katrina. He also conducted more than 30 field investigations while working for several years as a Medical Officer for CDC, NIOSH. Dr. Miller received his M.D. from Rush Medical College in Chicago, Illinois and his M.P.H. in environmental and occupational health sciences from the University of Illinois School of Public Health. He is board certified in occupational and environmental medicine. He is a member of APHA, American College of Occupational and En-vironmental Medicine, and American Conference of Governmental Industrial Hygienists.

Faith Mitchell, Ph.D., is President and CEO of Grantmakers In Health (www.gih.org), the Washington, DC–based philanthropic affinity group that supports and informs the work of health foundations and corporate giving programs. A national organization, GIH works with hundreds of health funders across the country. From 2007 to 2012, Dr. Mitchell was Vice President for Program and Strategy at GIH. Throughout her career, she has bridged research, practice, and policy to improve population health. She served 12 years at the National Academies, both at the IOM, where she was responsible for the health disparities portfolio, and as a Center Director in the Division of Social and Behavioral Sciences and Education. At the National Academies, she coedited several major reports on topics that included urban governance, racial/ethnic trends, and health disparities. She has also held leadership positions at the U.S. Department of State, The William and Flora Hewlett Foundation, and The San Francisco Foundation. Dr. Mitchell serves on numerous boards related to improving health and health care. She holds a doctorate in medical anthropology from UC Berkeley.

Lori Peek, Ph.D., is Associate Professor of Sociology and Codirector of the Center for Disaster and Risk Analysis at Colorado State University. She is also an Adjunct Research Scientist at the National Center for Disaster Preparedness at Columbia University. She is currently involved in several research projects, including a participatory project on children's recovery after the Joplin tornado and the Slave Lake wildfires; a 5-year project on the potential mental and physical health effects of the BP oil spill on children; a study of risk perception and evacuation behavior in hurricane-prone communities along the U.S. Gulf and Atlantic coasts; a global examination of earthquake risk reduction activities; and a statewide survey of disaster preparedness among child care providers in Colorado. She is the Co-founder and Co-director, along with Dr. David Abramson of the SHOREline disaster recovery and youth empowerment program. Dr. Peek has published widely on vulnerable populations and the sociology of disasters. She is author of *Behind the Backlash: Muslim Americans After 9/11*, co-author of *Children of Katrina*, and co-editor of *Displaced: Life in the Katrina Diaspora*. Dr. Peek received the Distinguished Book Award from the Midwest Sociological Society in 2012 and the Best Book Award from the American Sociological Association Section on Altruism, Morality, and Social Solidarity in 2013. In 2009, the American Sociological Association Section on Children and Youth honored her with its Early Career Award for Outstanding Scholarship.

Sally Phillips, R.N., Ph.D., has been serving as Acting Principal Deputy Assistant Secretary within the U.S. Department of Homeland Security (DHS) Office of Health Affairs (OHA) since May 2013. Dr. Phillips joined DHS in August 2010 and served as the Deputy Director of the Health Threats Resilience Division until March 2012, when she was promoted to the Deputy Assistant Secretary and Director of the Health Threats Resilience Division. Dr. Phillips provides leadership and direction to five major programmatic areas within OHA: biological and chemical defense; food, agriculture, and veterinary defense; planning and exercise support; health incidence surveillance; and state and local initiatives. Under her leadership, the department strengthened the biodefense enterprise through guidance for medical countermeasures and management of the BioWatch Program and National Biosurveillance Integration Center. Furthermore during this time, OHA saw increased funding and support of Congress for chemical defense programs; revised plans for disaster response support to FEMA; and development of guidance for radiation and nuclear disasters. Dr. Phillips comes to OHA from HHS, Agency for Healthcare Research and Quality (AHRQ) where she served as Director of the Public Health Emergency Preparedness Research Program. In July 2009 she joined the HHS Office of the ASPR as a Senior Advisor. There she was involved in policy issues, primarily supporting the H1N1 Task Force by addressing medical surge capacity and policies related to health care systems' preparedness and response to H1N1. Dr. Phillips is a leader in health system surge capacity and emergency preparedness. In her role at AHRQ, she served on numerous agency and department workgroups concerned with public health and medical response as well as homeland security preparedness and response initiatives. She is an accomplished author, consultant, and speaker on public health, medical preparedness, and response research initiatives. She also has expertise in health professional education and professional practice policy. Prior to joining AHRQ, Dr. Phillips was a Robert Wood Johnson Foundation Health Policy Fellow and Health Policy Analyst for Senator Tom Harkin for 2 years. She has also had a distinguished academic career in the Schools of Nursing and Medicine at the University of Colorado Health Sciences Center. She received a bachelor's degree from Ohio State University, a master's degree from the University of Colorado, and a doctorate from Case Western Reserve University. Her primary area of clinical practice is the care of women, infants, and children, with a specialty in the care of high-risk neonates.

Steven Phillips, M.D., is the Director, Specialized Information Services, and Associate Director, National Library of Medicine (NLM), NIH, HHS. He is leading the effort to establish a Disaster Information Management Research Center at NLM. This center, totally devoted to disaster health information and informatics, is the first of its kind in the world. Dr. Phillips is a graduate of Hobart College and Tufts Medical School. He is board certified both in general and thoracic surgery. Prior to coming to NIH, he lived in Des Moines, Iowa, where he practiced cardiac surgery. Dr. Phillips was a member of the Board of Regents of NLM from 1993 to 1997 and the 1997 Board Chair. From 1999 to 2001, He served as the full-time Deputy to the Director for Research and Education at the NLM, NIH. He served twice in Vietnam and retired from the U.S. Army Reserve as a Lieutenant Colonel in 1993. He is a life member of the 101st Airborne Associations and an associate life member of the UDT-SEAL Association. He sits on the Board of the Vietnam Veterans Memorial Reception Center, and serves as a member of a congressionally mandated DoD Wounded Warriors Task Force. He is Past President of the American Society for Artificial Internal Organs, the Society of Cardiac Surgeons of Spain, and of the Polk County Medical Society, Iowa. He has numerous publications, including approximately 125 in peer-reviewed medical journals, and has been granted 6 patents.

David Prezant, M.D., is the Chief Medical Officer for the Fire Department of the City of New York (FDNY) and the Special Advisor to the Fire Commissioner for Health Policy. He is FDNY's senior Pulmonary Consultant, Codirector of FDNY's WTC Medical Programs, and the PI for the NIOSH-funded FDNY WTC Data Center. He is also Professor of Medicine at the Albert Einstein College of Medicine, Director of their pulmonary medicine course for second year medical students, and a pulmonary physician at their main teaching hospital, Montefiore Medical Center. Dr. Prezant received his bachelor of Science from Columbia College in 1977 and his doctor of medicine from the Albert Einstein College of Medicine in 1981. After completing his internal medicine residency at Harlem Hospital, he returned to Albert Einstein College of Medicine and Montefiore Medical Center in New York for his pulmonary fellowship training. Dr. Prezant was instrumental in the development and design of the IAFF Wellness Fitness Initiative and the IAFF Candidate Physical Ability Test. Prior to 9/11/01, his research led to a better understanding of the impact of firefighting protective gear on burn injuries, smoke inhalation, and physical performance. On 9/11/01, Dr. Prezant was at the WTC taking care of FDNY firefighters and EMS rescue workers. He was present during the collapse and the aftermath and helped with triage efforts. Since that day he has devoted his entire clinical and research efforts to (1) the design and implementation of a medical monitoring and treatment program for FDNY firefighters and EMS WTC rescue workers funded by FDNY and NIOSH and (2) improvements in EMS prehospital medical care. To date, Dr. Prezant has published nearly 50 research papers on the health impact of WTC Collapse on NYC firefighters and EMS workers including papers in the *New England Journal of Medicine*, *The Lancet,* CDC's *Morbidity and Mortality Weekly Report*, *Environmental Health Perspectives*, the *American Journal of Respiratory and Critical Care Medicine* and *Chest*. This work has been instrumental in identifying WTC-related illnesses such as asthma, chronic bronchitis, bronchiolitis, rhinosinusitis, vocal cord dysfunction, gastroesophageal reflux, mental health disturbances, and cancers. In recognition of these activities, Dr. Prezant is a member of the International Association of Fire Fighters Redmond Advisory Board and the National Fire Protection Association Health and Safety Committee (co-author of NFPA 1582: Standard on Comprehensive Occupational Medical Program for Fire Departments), as well as a recipient of the American Thoracic Society's Public Service Award (2011) and the American College of Chest Physicians' Presidential Citation Honor Lecture (2012).

Irwin Redlener, M.D., founded and directs the National Center for Disaster Preparedness (NCDP) at Columbia University's Earth Institute. He is also Professor of Health Policy and Management at the Mailman School of Public Health and Professor of Pediatrics in the College of Physicians and Surgeons at Columbia University. Dr. Redlener is recognized as one of the nation's leading experts on preparing for, responding to, and recovering from large-scale disasters. He has written and spoken widely on disaster resiliency and vulnerability of special populations, with a special interest in the impact of disasters on children. He recently served as a commissioner on the federally legislated National Commission on Children and Disasters.

Dr. Redlener and his team have done seminal research on recovery, nuclear terrorism, and other catastrophic events. NCDP has followed families affected by major disasters including 9/11, Hurricane Katrina, the flooding of New Orleans, and the Deepwater Horizon oil spill. The center has also worked with officials following the devastating tornadoes that struck Joplin, Missouri. Dr. Redlener has also led major analyses of the risks associated with major pandemics, policies related to the preparedness for nuclear terrorism, and factors that influence public readiness for disasters in general. He has worked extensively with key officials in federal agencies and the White House. Dr. Redlener is also Co-founder (with Paul Simon) and President of the Children's Health Fund (CHF), established in 1987 to provide comprehensive health care to some of the nation's most medically underserved children. CHF currently supports mobile pediatric clinics serving disadvantaged children in urban and rural communities across the United States. CHF, in partnership with NCDP, has deployed mobile clinics providing medical care in the immediate aftermath of Hurricane Andrew (1992, Florida), the 9/11 attacks, Hurricane Katrina (Gulf, 2005) and the Deepwater Horizon crisis (2010), as well as responding immediately to care for victims of Hurricane Sandy in New York and New Jersey. Dr. Redlener is the author of *Americans at Risk: Why We Are Not Prepared for Megadisasters and What We Can Do Now* (Knopf, 2006).

Ellen Schenk, M.P.H., is currently a Fellow with both the Office of Emergency Medical Services with the National Highway Traffic Safety Administration (NHTSA) and the Emergency Medical Services for Children Program with the Health Resources and Services Administration (HRSA). With NHTSA and HRSA, Ms. Schenk has contributed to projects of national significance in the areas of emergency preparedness, research, and regionalization of care. Prior to the fellowship, Ms. Schenk's professional background was in global health, having worked to strengthen injury and emergency care systems in Malaysia, Mozambique, and several countries in Latin America. Ms. Schenk holds a bachelor of science in molecular and cell biology and Spanish from the University of Illinois at Urbana-Champaign as well as a master's degree in public health from Emory University. She will be continuing her studies this fall in the health systems doctoral program within the International Health Department of the Johns Hopkins Bloomberg School of Public Health.

Paul J. Seligman, M.D., M.P.H., is Executive Director for Global Regulatory Policy at Amgen. Prior to joining Amgen in 2012, he had a 28+ year public health career in the federal government. At FDA, he served as the Director of FDA's Latin America Regional Office, the Associate Director for Safety Policy and Communication in the Center for Drug Evaluation and Research (CDER), and the Director of the Office of Pharmacoepidemiology and Statistical Science. Before joining FDA in July 2001, Dr. Seligman served for 7 years as the Deputy Assistant Secretary for

Health Studies at the Department of Energy. He began his Public Health Service (PHS) career in 1983 at CDC as an Epidemic Intelligence Service officer. He completed a primary care internal medicine residency at the Cambridge Hospital in Cambridge, Massachusetts, prior to joining CDC. From 1974 to 1976, he was a Peace Corps volunteer in Kenya. Dr. Seligman holds an M.D. degree from UC, Davis, an M.P.H. in industrial health from the University of Michigan, and a B.S. in chemistry from Yale University. He is board certified in internal medicine, occupational medicine, and public health and general preventive medicine. He is a retired Commissioned Officer from the USPHS, having attained the rank of Rear Admiral.

Craig Slatin, Sc.D., M.P.H., is Professor of Health Education and Policy in the Department of Community Health and Sustainability, College of Health Sciences, University of Massachusetts Lowell. He is the PI and Director of The New England Consortium, an awardee of the NIEHS Worker Education and Training Program. Dr. Slatin's research has addressed health and safety training evaluation, occupational health disparities, and the political economy of the work environment. He has published peer-reviewed articles, editorials and commentaries, book chapters, and a book titled *Environmental Unions: Labor and the Superfund* (2009, Baywood Publishing Company, Inc.). Dr. Slatin is the editor of *New Solutions: A Journal of Environmental and Occupational Health Policy* (Baywood Publishing), which strives to bring together academic researchers, advocates, and activists. He has been an Occupational Health Investigator for the Massachusetts Department of Labor and Industries and an Environmental Health Inspector for the City of Boston Health Department. He is an active member of his own union, the Massachusetts Teachers' Association.

Anthony H. Speier, Ph.D., holds an appointment as Associate Professor in the Department of Psychiatry at Louisiana State University Health Sciences Center. Dr. Speier serves as Senior Project Leader for the Mental and Behavioral Health Capacity Project, which is developing sustainable integrated health care models in response to the health impact of the BP oil spill in the Gulf of Mexico. In November 2013 Dr. Speier retired from his position as Assistant Secretary for the Louisiana Office of Behavioral Health after 33 years of state service. He is a developmental psychologist and the former Assistant Secretary of the Louisiana Office of Behavioral Health. In his appointed position as Assistant Secretary, he has functioned as the State Authority for Mental Health and Substance Use Disorders. He has significant experience directly managing large and complex health systems–level budgets and assuring compliance with all state and federal regulatory and grant-specific reporting and operational responsibilities. Dr. Speier has served as the PI on numerous federal disaster response grants, including the $100 million Hurricane Katrina response, which he managed via the principles of a community-based participatory model. Dr. Speier has directed many crisis response programs, most recently, the Substance Abuse and Mental Health Services Administration SERG grant, which was an innovative multi-state crisis response collaborative across the Gulf states of Lousiana, Mississippi, and Alabama.

Holly A. Taylor, M.P.H., Ph.D., is currently Associate Professor in the Department of Health Policy and Management, Johns Hopkins Bloomberg School of Public Health, and a Core Faculty member of the Johns Hopkins Berman Institute of Bioethics. She received her B.A. from Stanford University, her M.P.H. from the School of Public Health at the University of Michigan, and her Ph.D. in health policy with a concentration in bioethics from the Johns Hopkins Bloomberg School of Public Health. Before pursuing her doctoral degree, Dr. Taylor was a Presidential Management Intern with the Department of Health and Human Services and spent 2 years as Special Assistant to the Director of the National Institute of Allergy and Infectious Diseases, NIH. Dr. Taylor offers a course on ethics in public health and health care policy. Her primary research interests are research ethics, local implementation of federal policy relevant to human subject research, civilian biodefense, and HIV/AIDS policy.

Robert J. Ursano, M.D., is widely published in the areas of posttraumatic stress disorder and public health planning for the psychological effects of terrorism, bioterrorism, traumatic events, and disasters including war. Dr. Ursano has more than 300 publications, is the co-author or editor of 8 books and is editor of *Psychiatry: Interpersonal and Biological Processes* and senior editor of the first *Textbook of Disaster Psychiatry* (Cambridge University Press), which was published in 2007. He was the first Chairman of the American Psychiatric Association's Committee on Psychiatric Dimensions of Disaster. Dr. Ursano chaired the development of the first American Psychiatric Association's Treatment Practice Guidelines for the Treatment of Patients with Acute Stress Disorder and Posttraumatic Stress Disorder. He has received the U.S. Department of Defense Humanitarian Service Award and the highest award of the International Traumatic Stress

Society, The Lifetime Achievement Award, for "outstanding and fundamental contributions to understanding traumatic stress." He is the recipient of the William C. Porter Award from the Association of Military Surgeons of the United States.

Dennis Wenger, Ph.D., is Program Director for program element 1638, Infrastructure Systems Management and Extreme Events, at the National Science Foundation (NSF). He had previously been at NSF from 2001 to 2005. Dr. Wenger was at Texas A&M University from 1989 to 2007. At Texas A&M, where he was a Professor of Urban and Regional Science and an Adjunct Professor of Sociology. He was also the Founding Director and Senior Scholar of the Hazard Reduction & Recovery Center. Prior to his arrival at Texas A&M in 1989, Dr. Wenger was on the faculty of the University of Delaware, where he served as Co-director of the Disaster Research Center from 1984 to 1989. Dr. Wenger has been engaged in research on hazards and disasters for more than 40 years. His research has focused on the social and multidisciplinary aspects of natural, technological, and human-induced disasters. Specifically, he has studied such topics as local emergency management capabilities and response, police and fire planning and response to disasters, search and rescue and the delivery of emergency medical services, mass media coverage of disasters, warning systems and public response, factors related to local community recovery success, and disaster beliefs and emergency planning. He undertook the only empirical study of the evacuation of the WTC towers after the first terrorist attack in 1993 and served as the PI for the first project to Enable the Future Generation of Hazard Researchers. He is the author of numerous books, research monographs, articles, and papers. Dr. Wenger currently serves as Chair of the United Nations Scientific and Technical Advisory Group to the International Strategy for Disaster Reduction. At NSF, Dr. Wenger serves as the foundation's representative to the Subcommittee on Disaster Reduction (SDR), which is associated with the OSTP of the White House. Dr. Wenger serves as Co-chair of the SDR.

Gamunu Wijetunge, M.P.M., NREMT-P, currently serves as the lead staff member for preparedness and workforce issues in the National Highway Traffic Safety Administration's (NHTSA's) Office of Emergency Medical Services. Mr. Wijetunge came to NHTSA in November 2001 after working as a paramedic in Bethesda, Maryland. His responsibilities at NHTSA involve a broad range of preparedness issues including pandemic influenza and integration of preparedness into the day-to-day EMS system.

His work involves close coordination with a number of federal agency partners through the Federal Interagency Committee on EMS. Mr. Wijetunge holds a master's degree in public management from the University of Maryland's School of Public Policy and is a member of the public administration academic honor society, Pi Alpha Alpha. He also holds a bachelor of science in emergency health services from the University of Maryland Baltimore County. He serves as President of the Wheaton Volunteer Rescue Squad, where he has volunteered since 1995 and is an actively practicing paramedic/firefighter holding the rank of Captain.

Howard A. Zucker, M.D., J.D., L.L.M., is First Deputy Commissioner of Health for the state of New York. In his present role he oversees preparedness issues as they relate to health care and is also focused on issues of hospital restructuring, elder care, and research aspects of medical marijuana. He has served as Assistant Director-General of the World Health Organization, Deputy Assistant Secretary of Health at HHS, White House Fellow, and Harvard Kennedy School Institute of Politics Fellow. He is Professor of Clinical Anesthesiology at Albert Einstein College of Medicine and Senior Advisor in the Division of Global Health & Human Rights at Massachusetts General Hospital. He created and led the nation's Medical Reserve Corps, which presently has more than 200,000 volunteers. Dr. Zucker has worked on Capitol Hill during the anthrax crisis, integrally involved with responses to SARS, H5N1, H1N1, and intellectual property aspects of pharmaceuticals during disasters. He has served as a public health expert for NATO and taught bioterrorism law. Dr. Zucker trained in pediatrics at Johns Hopkins, in anesthesiology at the Hospital of the University of Pennsylvania, pediatric anesthesiology/critical care at Children's Hospital of Philadelphia, and pediatric cardiology at Children's Hospital Boston. He has served as Director of the Intensive Care Unit at New York Presbyterian Hospital and held faculty appointments at Columbia, Cornell, Yale, NIH, and Georgetown. Dr. Zucker received his M.D. from George Washington University Medical School, J.D. from Fordham University Law School, and L.L.M. from Columbia Law School.

E

Speakers and Registered Attendees

David Abramson
National Center for Disaster Preparedness

Joie Acosta
RAND Corporation

Terry Adirim
Health Resource Services Administration/U.S. Dept. of Health and Human Services

Kathy Ahlmark
National Institute of Environmental Health Sciences

Nell Allbritton
Louisiana Department of Health and Hospitals

Brian Altman
National Center for Disaster Medicine and Public Health

Stacey Arnesen
National Library of Medicine/National Institutes of Health

Erik Auf der Heide
Centers for Disease Control and Prevention/Agency for Toxic Substance Disease Registry

Judith Bader
U.S. Dept. of Health and Human Services/Assistant Secretary for Preparedness and Response

Michael Baker
MDB, Inc.

Gerrit Bakker
Association of State and Territorial Health Officials

John Balbus
National Institute of Environmental Health Sciences

Joseph Barbera
George Washington University/Institute for Crisis, Disaster, and Risk Management

Anthony Barone
U.S. Dept. of Health and Human Services/Assistant Secretary for Preparedness and Response

Martha Bartz
National Disaster Medical System

Sharon Beard
National Institute of Environmental Health Sciences/Worker Education and Training Program

Georges C. Benjamin
American Public Health Association

April Bennett
National Institute of Environmental Health Sciences

Jeffrey Bethel
Oregon State University

Paul Biddinger
Massachusetts General Hospital/Dept. of Emergency Medicine

Linda Birnbaum
National Institutes of Health

Marvin Birnbaum
World Association for Disaster and Emergency Medicine

Daniel Bond
University of Southern Mississippi

Stephen Bradberry
Alliance Institute, Inc.

Shayne Brannman
Assistant Secretary for Preparedness and Response/Office of Emergency Management/ U.S. Dept. of Health and Human Services

Patricia Bright
U.S. Geological Survey

Chris Brown
Occupational Safety and Health Administration

Jeremy Brown
National Institutes of Health

Linda Brown
RTI International

Patrick Byrne

Charles B. Cairns
University of North Carolina/Dept. of Emergency Medicine

Amanda Carruth
Louisiana Public Health Institute

Shion Chang
Infectious Diseases Society of America

Seung-Hyun Cho
RTI International

Franco Ciammachilli
U.S. Dept. of Health and Human Services/Assistant Secretary for Preparedness and Response

Norman Coleman
U.S. Dept. of Health and Human Services/Assistant Secretary for Preparedness and Response

Francis Collins
National Institutes of Health/National Institute of Environmental Health Sciences

Gwen Collman
National Institutes of Health/ Extramural Research and Training

Ashley Conley
City of Nashua, New Hampshire Division of Public Health and Community Services

Rebecca Costello
Loudoun County Medical Response Corps

Mary Pat Couig
U.S. Department of Veteran, Affairs

Brooke Courtney
U.S. Food and Drug Administration

Hillary Craddock
National Center for Disaster Medicine and Public Health

Sharon Croisant
University of Texas Medical Branch

Kathleen Danskin
U.S. Dept. of Health and Human Services/Assistant Secretary for Preparedness and Response

Timothy Davis
U.S. Dept. of Health and Human Services/Assistant Secretary for Preparedness and Response/Office of Emergency Management/National Disaster Medical System

Lisa Delaney
National Institute for Occupational Safety and Health

Diane DiEuliis
Office of the Assistant Secretary for Preparedness and Response

Aram Dobalian
U.S. Department of Veterans Affairs

Daniel Dodgen
U.S. Dept. of Health and Human Services/Assistant Secretary for Preparedness and Response

Darrin Donato
U.S. Dept. of Health and Human Services/Assistant Secretary for Preparedness and Response

Brendan Doyle
U.S. Environmental Protection Agency/Office of Research and Development/National Homeland Security Research Center

Shelley DuTeaux
California Department of Public Health

Suzanne Dykstra
Center for Truth, Justice and Healing

Aaron Eagan
North Florida/South Georgia Veterans Health Administration

Betsy Eagin
MDB, Inc.

Bradley Eckert
Institute of Medicine

Donald Ellenberger
Center for Protection of Workers' Rights

Tom Fitzgerald
National Center for Disaster Medicine and Public Health

Shira Flax
U.S. Dept. of Homeland Security

Michael Focazio
U.S. Geological Survey

Patricia Fullam
Fire Department of the City of New York

Sandro Galea
Columbia University Mailman School of Public Health

Kiza Gates
U.S. Geological Survey

Jane Gelbmann
U.S. Dept. of Health and Human Services/Assistant Secretary for Financial Resources

Michael J. Gill
National Institutes of Health/National Library of Medicine/Lister Hill National Center for Biomedical Communications/Communications Engineering Branch

Lewis R. Goldfrank
New York University School of Medicine/Dept. of Emergency Medicine

Bernard D. Goldstein
University of Pittsburgh School of Public Health/Dept. of Environmental and Occupational Health

Michael Gottesman
National Institutes of Health/ Intramural Research

Natalie Grant
U.S. Dept. of Health and Human Services/Assistant Secretary for Preparedness and Response/Office of Emergency Management

Lynn Grattan
University of Maryland School of Medicine

Caitlin Greenbaum
Harvard School of Public Health

Samuel Groseclose
Office of Public Health Preparedness and Response/Centers for Disease Control and Prevention

Elin Gursky
Analytic Services, Inc.

Chanelle Gutari
George Washington University/ Institute for Crisis, Disaster and Risk Management

James Guyton
A.T. Kearney

Chris Hafner-Eaton
National Institutes of Health/Foundation for Advanced Education in the Sciences/Graduate Public Health Department

Pertt I. Hakkinen
National Institutes of Health/ National Library of Medicine

Cynthia Hansen
U.S. Dept. of Health and Human Services/Assistant Secretary for Preparedness and Response

Theresa Harris
American Association for the Advancement of Science

Jack Herrmann
National Association of County and City Health Officials

Michael Heumann
Heumann Health Consulting
Council of State and Territorial Epidemiologists (consultant)

Kevin Horahan
U.S. Dept. of Health and Human Services/Assistant Secretary for Preparedness and Response

John Howard
Centers for Disease Control and Prevention/National Institute for Occupational Safety and Health

Sandra Howard
U.S. Dept. of Health and Human Services

Marilyn Howarth
Center of Excellence in Environmental Toxicology/University of Pennsylvania

Joseph "Chip" Hughes
National Institute of Environmental Health Sciences/Worker Education and Training Branch

Jean Hu-Primmer
U.S. Food and Drug Administration/Office of Chief Scientists/Office of Counterterrorism and Emerging Threats

Karen Huss
National Institutes of Health/National Institute of Nursing Research

Angel Ip
Association of School and Programs of Public Health/U.S. Environmental Protection Agency

David Jett
National Institutes of Health/National Institute of Neurological Disorders and Stroke

Vikas Kapil
Agency for Toxic Substances Disease Registry/Centers for Disease Control and Prevention

Katherine Kirkland
Association of Occupational and Environmental Clinics

Deborah Knickerbocker
Office of Emergency Management/Assistant Secretary for Preparedness and Response/U.S. Dept. of Health and Human Services

Lisa Koonin
Centers for Disease Control and Prevention

Walter Koroshetz
National Institutes of Health

David L. Lakey
Texas Department of State Health Services

Jennifer Langhinrichsen-Rohling
Gulf Coast Behavioral Health and Resiliency Center

Adrianne Lazer
George Washington University School of Medicine

Joy Lee
MDB, Inc.

Mary Leinhos
Centers for Disease Control and Prevention

Lauren Lewis
Centers for Disease Control and Prevention

Maureen Lichtveld
Tulane School of Public Health and Tropical Medicine

Donald A. B. Lindberg
National Institutes of Health/ National Library of Medicine

Kenneth Lindemann

Rebecca Lipsitz
U.S. Food and Drug Administration

Sarah Lister
Congressional Research Service

Cindy Love
National Library of Medicine/Disaster Information Management Research Center

Maribeth Love
U.S. Dept. of Health and Human Services

Diana Luan
Center for Technology and National Security Policy/National Defense University

Kristin Ludwig
U.S. Geological Survey

Nicole Lurie
U.S. Dept. of Health and Human Services/Assistant Secretary for Preparedness and Response

Gary Machlis
Clemson University

Carmen Maher
Office of Counterterrorism and Emerging Threats/Office of the Chief Scientist/Office of the Commissioner/U.S. Food and Drug Administration

Bert Maidment
National Institutes of Health/National Institute of Allergy and Infectious Diseases

Josephine Malilay
National Center for Environmental Health/ Centers for Disease Control and Prevention

Eric Mangahis

Jenna Manheimer
Association of Schools and Programs and Public Health/U.S. Environmental Protection Agency

Mary Masters
Westat

Denise Matthews
Occupational Safety and Health Administration

Keely Maxwell
U.S. Environmental Protection Agency

Marcia McNutt
U.S. Geological Survey

Sharon Medcalf
University of Nebraska Medical Center/College of Public Health

Maura Merlis
U.S. Dept. of Health and Human Services/Office of the General Counsel

Aubrey Miller
National Institute of Environmental Health Sciences

Faith Mitchell
Grantmakers In Health

Felicia Monahan
Center for Disease and Humanitarian Assistance Medicine

Joshua Morganstein
Uniformed Services University of the Health Sciences

Meghan Mott
Institute of Medicine

Francesca Music
U.S. Dept. of Defense

Elizabeth Nathaniel
Analytic Services, Inc.

Amy Nevel

GiaLinh Nguyen
George Washington University

Tonya Nichols
U.S. Environmental Protection Agency

Roberto Javier Nicolalde
Nicolalde R&D LLC

Lula Odom
International Chemical Workers Union Consortium Training Center

Thomas Orfanos
Global Safety First LLC
Luis Ortiz-Echevarria
International Medical Corps

Joan Packenham
National Institute of Environmental Health Sciences/National Institutes of Health

Benita Panigrahi
National Center for Disaster Preparedness/Columbia University

Carol Parsons
National Institutes of Health

Glenn Paulson
George Washington University School of Public Health

Skip Payne
Office of the Surgeon General

Lori Peek
Colorado State University/Dept. of Sociology

Ray Pena

Steve Peterson
National Institutes of Health

Sally Phillips
U.S. Dept. of Homeland Security/Office of Health Affairs

Steven Phillips
National Institutes of Health/National Library of Medicine

Ron Piedrahita
U.S. Dept. of Health and Human Services/Assistant Secretary for Preparedness and Response

Geoffrey Plumlee
U.S. Geological Survey

Margaret Potter
University of Pittsburgh Graduate School of Public Health

David Prezant
Fire Department of the City of New York

Rachel Pruchno
New Jersey Institute for Successful Aging/Rowan University

Paul Pulliam
RTI International

Nishadi Rajapakse
National Institutes of Health/National Institute on Minority Health and Health Disparities

Steven Ramsey
Social and Scientific Systems, Inc.

Irwin Redlener
National Center for Disaster Preparedness

Megan Reeve
Institute of Medicine

Tim Rehner
University of Southern Mississippi

Les Reinlib
National Institute of Environmental Health Sciences

Jim Remington

Alex Repace
Institute of Medicine

Richard Rosselli
Social and Scientific Systems, Inc.

Ivan Rusyn
University of North Carolina

Elizabeth Sadove
U.S. Food and Drug Administration

Jennifer Sass
National Resources Defense Council

Ruth Ellen Schelhaus

Ellen Schenk
U.S. Dept. of Transportation/National Highway Traffic Safety Administration/Office of Emergency Medical Services

Toby Schonfeld
U.S. Environmental Protection Agency

Kenneth Schor
National Center for Disaster Medicine and Public Health

John Scott
Center for Public Service Communications

Stephen Scroggs
ValueOptions, Inc.

Paul Seligman
Amgen, Inc.

Annum Shaikh
International Medical Corps

Susan Sherman
U.S. Dept. of Health and Human Services

Mark Shimamoto
U.S. Global Change Research Program

Craig Slatin
University of Massachusetts Lowell

Theresa Smith
Office of Public Health Preparedness and Response/Division of State and Local Readiness/Centers for Disease Control and Prevention

Rishi Sood
New York City Department of Health & Mental Hygiene

Anthony Speier
Louisiana State University Health Sciences Center/Dept. of Psychiatry

Kristin Stevens

Kandra Strauss-Riggs
National Center for Disaster Medicine and Public Health

Daniela Stricklin
Applied Research Associates

Barbara Styrt

William Suk
National Institutes of Health/National Institute of Environmental Health Sciences

Blerta Sulhasi
School Based Psychological Services Program

Ana Szarfman
U.S. Food and Drug Administration

Victoria Ta
Center for Disaster and Humanitarian Assistance Medicine

Holly Taylor
John Hopkins Bloomberg School of Public Health

George Thomas
National Institutes of Health/National Library of Medicine/Lister Hill National Center for Biomedical Communications/Communications Engineering Branch

Wendy Marie Thomas
National Oceanic and Atmospheric Administration/National Weather Service

Claudia Thompson
National Institute of Environmental Health Sciences

Jonathan Thornburg
RTI International

Robert J. Ursano
Uniformed Services University of the Health Services/Dept. of Psychiatry

Luis Vazquez
International Chemical Workers Union Consortium Training Center

Michelle Vine

Lauren Walsh
National Center for Disaster Medicine and Public Health

Deborah Weinstock
MDB, Inc.

Christopher Weis
National Institute of Environmental Health Sciences

Dennis Wenger
National Science Foundation

Paula Whitacre
National Institute of Environmental Health Sciences

Jalonne White-Newsome
WE ACT for Environmental Justice

Gam Wijetunge
U.S. Dept. of Transportation/National Highway Traffic Safety Administration/Office of Emergency Medical Services

Ryan Winkelvoss
Assistant Secretary for Preparedness and Response/ U.S. Dept. of Health and Human Services

Beverly L. Wright
Dillard University

Marci Wright
U.S. Dept. of Health and Human Services

Sophia Yang
Office of the Surgeon General

Kevin Yeskey
MDB, Inc.

Carmen A. Young
American Red Cross

Yon Yu
Centers for Disease Control and Prevention

Howard Zucker
New York State Department of Health

F

Statement of Task

An ad hoc committee will organize a public workshop that will examine how to enable methodological and ethical public health and medical research on disaster preparedness, response, and recovery in parallel with and/or immediately following future emergencies. The committee will develop the workshop agenda, select and invite speakers and discussants, and moderate the discussions. Specifically, the workshop participants will

- Discuss how to ensure adequate protections for human research participants.
    - o Discuss principles that would strengthen informed consent during emergency use scenarios.
    - o Explore mechanisms to ensure that investigators and research institutions are aware of resources available to minimize administrative burden.
    - o Consider potential tools and guidance that could be developed to enable institutions to utilize central institutional review boards (IRBs).
- Consider the opportunities and challenges associated with establishing a "research first responder" team.
    - o Discuss the roles and responsibilities of the research team and how it can perform its functions without interfering with response efforts.

  - o Examine what funding mechanisms and infrastructure requirements are necessary to facilitate "research first responder" teams.
  - o Consider what triggers could be used to activate the research infrastructure and teams.
- Consider opportunities and structures necessary to enable citizen scientists.

An individually authored summary of the presentations and discussions at the workshop will be prepared by a designated rapporteur in accordance with institutional guidelines.